FROM MEASLES TO MAGIC

Memoirs of a Medical Officer in Northern Nigeria 1957-1964

Kathleen Abraham

This First Edition published 2010 by
2QT Limited (Publishing)
Dalton Lane, Burton In Kendal
Cumbria LA6 1NJ

Cover Design by Robbie Associates
Cover Images supplied by the Author

Printed in Great Britain by
the MPG Books Group, Bodmin and King's Lynn

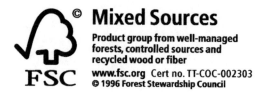

A CIP catalogue record for this book is available
from the British Library
ISBN 9781908098030

Dedication

This book has been written in memory of my husband.
It is dedicated to my children.
It comes too with a tip of the cap to all the friends, colleagues, and
patients, African and expatriate alike, from my time in Northern Nigeria.

Acknowledgements

My thanks are firstly due to the Editor of the British Medical Journal for permission to re-tell the story that appeared as a filler 'The Arrow that flieth by Day', in the BMJ of 15 April 1995.

I must also thank three people who gallantly read and commented on the book when I had finished writing it. They are firstly, Barbara Telfer, a friend of many years; secondly, Dr David Elliott, my GP, who is a friend to all his patients; and lastly, Ray Underwood, who was the Principal of the Provincial Boys' Secondary School, Maiduguri, Northern Nigeria, during our time there. Not only did Ray read the manuscript, but he also provided the foreword. I am grateful to the Publisher 2QT for the helpful advice they have given to me.

My son and daughter have given much encouragement, and my son in particular has more than once rescued computer-illiterate me from the terrors of the keyboard. Furthermore, not only has he edited the manuscript with great care, but he has also spent many hours scanning the photographs that I selected for reproduction, ensuring that they were in good order. My thanks to both my children.

I have, so far as I know, preserved confidentiality where appropriate. If anyone feels that I have identified them when I should not have done, I sincerely apologise.

I never knew which of the guests at our wedding took the photograph of my husband and me in the church. I hope that whoever it was will not object to seeing it here. Thank you for taking it all those years ago. I myself took all the other photographs seen in this book.

Finally, apart from confidentiality, I have deliberately not mentioned names of more than one or two friends and colleagues from my overseas days. The reason for this is that there were so many, and strings of names during the memoir would become, I think, confusing to readers who had not been part of the communities there. I have only to look at the pages of signatures of those who attended our wedding, or re-read letters from friends we made in different stations, or recall chance meetings here and there during journeys, to remember how much Rex and I, separately and together, appreciated the friendship given to us. You all know who you are, and the fact that your names are not here doesn't mean that any of you slipped off our radar.

Foreword

These days, it seems, we are forever being asked to apologise for things done or left undone years and years ago, particularly with reference to our former colonies. Whether we, as the former power in Nigeria, gained more from our involvement with Nigeria than it did from us is not the concern of this foreword. This foreword seeks to celebrate, indirectly, the work of hundreds of British teachers, doctors, engineers, administrators and so on, who took the 'service' element of their appointment to the Colonial Service very seriously indeed.

Read this account of Dr Abraham's work in the far north of Nigeria and you will be left in no doubt about the unstinting help she gave, together with Dr Gonzales, not just to the local population of Maiduguri, but to people throughout the vast area of Bornu. You will discover the nature of the work done by Government medical officers not only in provincial headquarters, but also in outreach activities such as bush dispensaries throughout the province. In the course of 'one revolving moon' these doctors had to look after the Provincial hospital, and act also as GP, surgeon, physician, primary health care expert, midwife, visitor to local prisons, lunatic asylums and outlying dispensaries, and had to cope with anything else that called for medical expertise. In all this whirl of professional activity, Dr Abraham found time to meet the man who became her husband – whose own standards of service to the development of education were every bit as impressive as hers to health: he ran the Bornu Teacher Training College next door to the Provincial Boys' Secondary School of which I was the Principal.

Did Dr Abraham ever complain of being overworked or underpaid? Not to my knowledge. When she drove to the Provincial Secondary School with a proposal to open and run a school clinic, she was not planning to shed any of her other responsibilities. It seemed sensible to her to lay the foundations of good health in those being trained to run the country when the time came. Just another job to be done. Until then, our medical provision for some two hundred students consisted of three huge bottles of 'medicine' over which the Bursar presided, with, no doubt, back-up from the local dispensary. One was for problems above the belt. One was for problems below the belt. The third was for problems around the middle, for which a good knowledge of the local languages, Kanuri, Shuwa Arabic and Hausa, was a prerequisite. If he found himself out of his depth, the Bursar sent the boy off to the hospital with a request for a blood test. Would our boys, many well advanced into adulthood, mainly Moslem, and with a sense of modesty to a degree unheard of in English boarding schools, ever take to a lady doctor? I was sceptical. Well, they did, and thanks to Dr Abraham's blend of care with no-nonsense toughness, the queues to see her never got out of hand.

Even Manchester-trained doctors have their limitations, and I was pleased to see that Dr Abraham had to concede greater expertise to the old Kanuri lady who sat outside the canteens in town. The Bursar used to send boys suffering from a disease peculiar to Kanuris to me before they were allowed to go to see this 'wise woman'. All these Kanuri boys were quite convinced that sheer weight of learning was pressing on the roof of the mouth. A boy would shuffle into my office and tell me '*Kalanyi sukkuruna*' – 'My head has fallen'. A Kanuri problem, a Kanuri solution. Off he would go, cross the palm of the old lady with silver, and she would then thrust two rather grubby thumbs into his mouth and push its roof back into place. Fallen heads apart, Dr Abraham was each boy's personal physician, and they thought she was wonderful.

As you read these memoirs, you would do well to remember that her story is essentially that of many, if not most, Colonial Service officers. Fate guided her to the Colonial Office, and assigned her to a post in Northern Nigeria, a country about which she could have had very little foreknowledge. She couldn't have been prepared for the searing temperatures before and after the rains, or the dust-laden Harmattan wind that cracked the lips and blotted out the sun for days on end. She could never have imagined the market in Maiduguri through which her cook would have had to fight against a flystorm to get the meat for her dinner. No air-conditioning, temperamental kerosene fridges whose lamps were forever going out, sending plumes of acrid smoke billowing up to the ceiling, erratic water and electricity supplies.

Why, in retrospect, did we put up with it all for so long?

Dr Abraham's memoir tells us why, and shows how it is that so many of us look back on the years of service in the colonies as amongst the most rewarding of our lives.

Raymond Underwood
Served in the Education Department of Northern Nigeria from 1954 until the mid 1960s. He was Principal of the Provincial Boys Secondary School, Maiduguri during the time of the School Medical Service, later being posted to Kaduna as Inspector of English.

Preface

This is an account of the years I spent as a medical officer in the Overseas Civil Service in Northern Nigeria. Much will, inevitably, have changed now in Nigeria, and I have felt for some time that it might be of interest to record the life there of a general duties medical officer in the late nineteen fifties – early sixties. That was, of course, in the immediate pre and post Independence years. I have also tried to give a picture of my life as an expatriate among people whose various cultures were so different from my own.

It has been fun to write this book, albeit tinged with nostalgia, even sadness now and again. I have re-lived many wonderful times while setting everything down on paper. There has been great pleasure in retrieving all the memories, and in re-reading all the letters that I had sent home which, unknown to me, had been kept by my parents, and from some of which I have quoted verbatim here. If I had my time all over again, I would do exactly the same thing. I have never regretted writing to the Colonial Office to ask if there were any jobs going in Africa for doctors.

Kathleen Abraham
Caton 2010

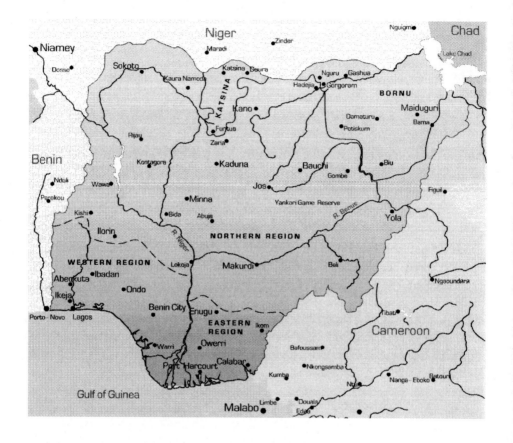

A map of Nigeria showing towns and cities mentioned in the book. Approximate positions are also indicated for the former regional boundaries (dotted lines) and the Bornu and Katsina provincial boundaries (solid lines) as they were in 1962.

Outset

"That's Africa," said a voice behind me.

I turned round from the ship's rail to see who had spoken.

There stood one of the 'old coasters', one of my shipmates, who was returning from leave. He smiled and pointed across the sea to the east, where there was a blackness just above the horizon that was something other than salt water. Little points of light flickered here and there on it, and it was tinged with the last rays of the setting sun behind us.

"That's Africa," repeated my companion, "Take a deep breath and you'll smell Africa. And you'll never forget it as long as you live."

I looked again across the sea to the dark mass, now grown a little larger, and I breathed in.

Sure enough, on the breeze there came the smell of a myriad things – of heat, sand, animals, earth, vegetation, wet dust after rain, people, the smoke of a thousand cooking fires – the smell of Africa. And I have indeed never forgotten it.

My pulse raced in anticipation of the moment, still a few days away, when I would set foot on this vast continent where I was to work as a medical officer in Northern Nigeria, a thousand miles up-country from Lagos, our port of disembarkation.

Chapter 1

I went out to work in Nigeria in 1957, shortly before Regional Independence, and I retired from overseas service at the end of 1964, a few years after full Federal Independence came to the country.

Those of us who were there then have been privileged to take part in a way of life that I suspect will no longer exist. As we all grow older, it seems fitting that some of us at least, write down as much as we can remember of those times. Colonialism has become an unacceptable word for some people, but I remember colonial servants being men and women of great integrity, and I also remember many of the Africans amongst whom I lived and worked expressing their apprehension about what would become of their country once we had all gone. Indeed there were some who did not want the British to leave.

Why did I go there anyway? I think on impulse as much as anything. During the ten years since I'd qualified, I'd had varied experience in several hospitals and many disciplines. The years had been extremely happy and seemed to go by in a flash. My chosen career felt more like a hobby for which I was actually being paid rather than a job of work done in order to make a living. This enjoyment remained right up to my final retirement.

However, I realised one day that I had reached a watershed. What to do next? The answer came by way of a doctor who had gone to work in Rhodesia and who had just come to the UK on leave. His description of his life and work overseas grabbed me. The seed was sown, and I wrote to the Colonial Office asking if there were any medical posts going in Africa. There were, and after sending in a completed application form, I was asked to attend for interview. My main memory of that day was of being conducted up flights of stairs and along dusty corridors before being ushered into a tiny room, more like a store-cupboard than anything else. When I had eased myself round the door I saw that in front of me was a baize covered table, behind which sat three gentlemen, with their backs up against the wall behind them and their tummies seemingly squashed against the table in front of them. There was a single chair at my side – for me – and I sat down. The interview was searching but non-committal. I was told that there was a post going in Northern Nigeria, and that in due course I would be written to and told whether or not it might be for me. A few days later a letter came to say that the job was mine if I wanted it, and would I tell them whether or not I would accept their offer. Of course I accepted. Somehow from the moment I had set foot in the Colonial Office and proceeded into the Dickensian atmosphere of the interview, it had seemed both 'right' and inevitable. Therefore whenever I am asked "Why did you choose Nigeria?" I always want to say, "I didn't. Nigeria chose me."

During the next few months, while I was continuing to earn a living with various locum posts, information began to arrive. My posting was to be to Maiduguri, the provincial capital of Bornu in the far north-east of the country. The medical officer in charge there, Dr Simpson, wrote to me to welcome me in advance. His wife also wrote, to give me a few tips on housekeeping – including the yardage of material I would need when making curtains for my house. She was spot on – when I finished there was only a six-inch strip of fabric left over.

Booklets arrived describing some features of Nigeria. A list of vaccinations and immunisations popped through the letterbox, with instructions to get myself 'done' with them all – yellow fever, typhoid, smallpox, but strangely nothing about polio. That was sharply remedied as soon as I arrived in the country however, for the first thing that happened was that I was given the injection with the words "There is a lot of polio here, so you go nowhere until you've had your shot" (polio vaccine was not given orally there in those days). Advice was also sent about malaria prophylaxis. In those days we had two alternatives – either a daily dose of Paludrine, or a twice weekly tablet of Nivaquine. I opted for Paludrine. One had to start taking anti-malarials a fortnight before going into an infected area, and continue for a month after returning to a temperate climate where the villainous mosquitoes were not found. Finally a book, 'Health and Hygiene in the Tropics' landed on the doormat, bound in bright green fabric and bearing the text 'This book has been treated with a poisonous insecticide'. I wonder if it is still despatched to would-be expatriate employees.

A nursing sister on leave in the UK contacted me to give me further information about what to expect. The trouble was that there was so much to be told that I remembered only little bits and had almost everything to learn when I got there.

I was lucky to obtain some lead lined chests for my chattels, having been told that lead linings were the only way of avoiding the ravages of marauding insects in the tropics. I bought as much in the way of basic equipment as I could, not knowing what I would be able to get hold of once in my station. Cooking utensils, bed-linen, table-linen, cutlery, crockery, books, ornaments, camping kit (I knew that I would probably do some bush touring), and clothes, all to be cotton, I had been told.

Most of the lead lined boxes have now been passed on to other people, but one remains with me, as does also my 'rot proof and insect proof' camp bed, together with its mosquito poles and net, all still as good as new. I also bought a tiny petrol stove, all of six or seven inches square, with which to cook meals when out on tour; and I acquired a miniature sewing machine as well, that looked like a toy but wasn't, and on that I made curtains for several different houses over the years as well as innumerable clothes. And I attended an abbreviated motor mechanics course in case I ever had to deal with car problems when out in the bush, while hoping desperately that I would never have a breakdown anywhere.

Finally my sailing date arrived. One was paid from the moment one left the home country en route for the overseas posting, so the voyage out (and I had never sailed before) was a bonus – a fortnight's delightful paid holiday. I watched the sea turn from a chill pewter to a soft translucent blue, and contemplated the lovely sights of flying fishes, and of dolphins playing round the ship. Having only had a few brief breaks since qualifying (young doctors were not paid very much in those days, and holidays did not come into the equation – one moved from one post to the next with no space in between), this journey was magical for me.

One of my cabin mates was a nursing sister returning from a sabbatical year. She was going to take charge of the Nurse Training School in Kano. She also tried to tell me something of what to expect. But nothing really prepared me for the actual experience.

I think, looking back, that what I remembered from what everyone tried to tell me were odd things like "Look out for thieves hooking all your possessions through the open windows" and, "You can order a year's supply of dry stores from Lagos and have it sent up-country to you". Nobody told me about the colour, the smells, the noise, the system, the protocols – the everyday stuff. I suppose all that was so normal to the old hands that they forgot it would be strange to me.

One evening, just as the sun was going down, we saw a black outline close to the eastern horizon – land! As the dusk deepened we could see little points of light here and there on the hillsides, with tiny plumes of smoke rising up into the sky. We were told that we were passing Dakar. For me this was the first sight of a strange, and to me unknown, continent in which, very soon, I would be living and working. It was an exhilarating moment. Suddenly the sea voyage, up to then an exciting experience for me, seemed mundane against what was to come. There, on the soft night air, something of Africa came across the water to steal my senses. I have never forgotten that moment.

The first port we put into was Freetown in Sierra Leone. Even when we were inshore, the sea still looked blue and was clear. The whole shoreline was very beautiful, with a wide sweep of the bay and a sandy beach fringed with palm trees. As we neared the dockside, I could see crowds of people there, all watching the ship come in. Gradually we came nearer and one could see individuals more clearly. I was intrigued by what I saw – the colour, the clothes, the mannerisms, the sheer apparent chaos. I saw women carrying their babies on their backs, tied on with long lengths of cloth. I saw how people carried everything on their heads, and commented in a letter home to my parents how I thought that because of the way in which head loads were carried, people had a very good deportment, but added that I thought all the women had hollow backs and protuberant bottoms because of the way in which they transported their babies.

I was amused to see one young child walking along with what looked for all the world like a small bottle of ink on her head – something I would carry in my hand. I was taken aback when I saw several men wearing in broad daylight what I took to be pyjamas – which seemed to me to be very odd. It was several days before I realised that what I was looking at was normal native dress – very sensibly made of cool cotton and constructed very loosely because of the hot climate. I was a real greenhorn!

As we were to spend several hours in Freetown so that the ship could take on supplies and deck passengers, and refuel, some of us shared a taxi and asked the driver to take us right round the town. We went past the old slave market with the huge cottonwood tree in its centre under which the slaves had been sold, then past the local canteens (the name given to the shops) – and up the hill behind the town centre, past the Government Residential Area. The hills behind gave a lovely backdrop to the town, and it was all very picturesque.

My nursing sister cabin mate tried all the time to tell me about the trees and flowers we passed – "Look, there's a jacaranda! – a paw-paw tree! – a Flame of the Forest tree!" – but we passed everything so quickly and it was all so new that I only had time to take in a general impression of lush foliage.

The houses in the Government Residential Area looked nice but much different from those back home. The dwellings in the town I thought of as 'shanties', and some would certainly merit the name, though many would not. Vultures were sitting on top of several houses, or flapping slowly and lazily round on a puff of wind, looking rather like big black ragged umbrellas. The town centre and the waterfront area looked rather seedy to my eyes, unaccustomed as yet to Africa. My mind whirled with the many impressions thrust upon it, especially when I dimly realised that before long, everything would start to become familiar to me.

I might point out here before going any further, that in those days in the UK, certainly in the smaller towns and villages, a coloured person was a rarity.

So most people I knew, including me, knew very little about Africans. I had personally only known one African – a Nigerian biochemist who worked in the Pathology lab at my hospital in Beverley. Even he would not be typical of the people amongst whom I would work, a thousand miles from Lagos and his part of the country.

All I had to go on, for any idea of Africa, was what I had been told by people I met on the ship going out – expatriates mostly who were returning from leave. I believed everything I was told and took everything at face value. As time went on I learnt by my own experiences and realised that sometimes what I had been told depended very much on the reaction of other people to situations, and that my own reactions were often very different.

I found that much depended upon one's own attitude and approaches, and also on one's manner of working. The Nigerians among whom I worked very soon knew who they considered to be a 'proper European'. They respected those who worked honestly and hard, and were quick to spot any sort of behaviour from an expatriate that they considered to be inappropriate.

An expatriate overseas could either work just according to the letter of his terms and conditions of service, or he could take his job seriously and throw himself into it and give 110% of himself to it and to the people among whom he was working. Most expatriates I knew were like this – we all worked hard, cared a lot about Nigeria, and put everything we had into our jobs. One vital quality was a sense of humour. If you couldn't laugh, then you had no business to be there.

Back on the boat we found that we had now taken on board a crowd of 'deck passengers' – local people who were travelling from Freetown to either Takoradi, our next port of call, in Ghana, or on to Lagos. I was fascinated by what I saw – a mass of people, some with their families, all with their belongings tied up in great bundles which had to be carried, usually as head loads. They catered for themselves and lived out on the open deck, for we were in the tropics and it was never cold, even the nights were soft and warm – even out at sea.

When we docked at Takoradi, and because again we were not to leave for several hours, once more some of us took a taxi ride around the town, and once more I was bemused by the sights and sounds that bombarded me. I was intrigued again to see how easily head loads were carried – and again remarked on the graceful and erect carriage of the women. You can't carry a head load if you don't walk evenly and keep your head high and steady.

Just before the ship tied up, and while we were slowly moving in to our berth, several small row boats came out to us, from which the boatmen would dive for coins which would be thrown from the ship for them. They sat on the sides of their little boats with one leg trailing in the water. Each eagle-eyed man would see the minute a coin was thrown, and immediately dived after it – you saw the diver go deep down, and you could see the coins in the water too, falling to the bottom. But every time, the money was caught and held before it had gone too far. The divers, I thought, deserved every penny they rescued. The exercise was lucrative for them and fascinating to watch.

When we returned to the ship it was all buttoned up and ready to go. Our cabins could be unlocked – we had been told to lock them firmly at Freetown and again at Takoradi, being informed that if we didn't, everything would be stolen by the time we got back to them – and shipboard life was resumed. We found that many deck passengers had disembarked and new ones had come aboard. An air of expectancy hovered over the whole ship as we got under way again for the last short leg of the journey. Our next stop would be Lagos. Those passengers who were returning to duty after leave began to talk to each other about their postings and gave each other messages to be delivered to friends in other stations. Newcomers like me wondered how long it would be before we in turn could call ourselves 'old coasters'. There were now only two of us in the cabin, as our third cabin-mate had left us at Takoradi. The cabin felt oddly empty without her – we had all three got on well together, but at the same time it gave the remaining two of us much more room in which to sort out our possessions and pack ready for Lagos.

I had enjoyed the voyage tremendously. It was, as I have said, in itself a new and exotic experience for me, in the course of which I had sometimes felt that I would like to sail on forever. The thought came into my mind that after my time in Nigeria I could do worse than go for a job as a ship's surgeon – why not? But for the moment I couldn't wait to reach Lagos and get stuck into my new post. The long process from deep sea to dockside seemed never ending a few days later, but finally the ship was tied up, the gangway opened to us and we disembarked. Whatever the fates had in store for me in Nigeria, here I was, and more than ready to find out.

Chapter 2

It was the last day of August when we arrived – the tail end of the rainy season. I told my parents in the first letter I sent home from Nigeria that it was not too warm a day, and that it was raining:

'31.8.57

You could have done as well at Bridlington. Anything less like the tropics you couldn't imagine at that moment... Lagos is much more of a town than Freetown, teeming with people, of course, in all stages of dress from nothing to Western styles. Most of them are barefoot. There are cars all over the place – very opulent, and flocks of goats and stray chickens on the roadside & sometimes in the road too. The smell is only bad in patches!'

Once off the boat, we were herded into the Customs shed. Our loads had already been taken there from the ship. I found mine eventually, and waited by them for somebody to come and check them. It looked as if it would be a long time, until I was approached by somebody who was obviously a rather senior policeman. He was English, and was in the uniform, as I later discovered, of the Federal police. "You waiting for the Customs men?" he asked me. "What's your name then?" I told him. "Where are you from, and what will you be doing here?" he asked. I told him – I was to work as a medical officer. I came from Hull and had been working in Beverley. "Good old Yorkshire!" was his reply, and he beckoned one of the Customs officers over to us. "Chalk this young lady through," he commanded. "She's a doctor, come to help your country, and she comes from Yorkshire where I come from, so she's all right!" he continued. The Customs officer laughed. "Good!" And he smiled and chalked me up without asking a single question as to what I might be bringing into the country.

Lagos I found to be a typical big bustling city – but one very different from any I had seen in Britain, for cheek by jowl with big buildings there were small houses, some even shanty-like. There were open drains in many of the streets and roadways, filled with all sorts of rubbish, and used openly as latrines by many people. We newly arrived ex-pats were amused to be told by the taxi driver who first took us to the Ikoyi Rest House that this was actually the first week in Lagos of traffic lights. He went on to say that most drivers –

of both public and private vehicles – were using other roads to get round the city, as they felt that these coloured lights were simply putting the evil eye on both vehicles and their drivers, and would therefore bring bad luck on them all. As I write this more than fifty years later, my recollections of that time in Lagos are still vivid, though not necessarily in chronological order.

One memory I have is how, after settling into our rooms at the Rest House, and having had our first meal there (lunch), I realised that most of my travelling companions were either drifting off to the bar for long cool drinks, or going back to their rooms for a long siesta. I didn't drink anything alcoholic in those days, nor did I want to rest on my bed. What I really wanted, after two weeks of relative inactivity on board ship was to stretch my legs and do something. To my surprise and pleasure, one of the people who had been on the ship said to me, "I don't want to spend the afternoon drinking and I really want to do something like going for a long walk. Would you like to come along? I'm sure we could explore a bit." Would I like that? Indeed I would. And off we set in the heat of the afternoon. We walked, it seemed, round the whole of Ikoyi, past big houses, small houses, over roads with a bit of tarmac, and over untarred roads, watched much of the time by the curious eyes of the local population who, very sensibly, were sitting in patches of shade. They must have thought we were quite mad, and probably we were. But I for one felt better after that couple of hours stretching my legs.

Later that evening, when the postprandial drift back to the bar began, my afternoon companion sought me out again. "How would you like another walk?" he asked, adding, "I really don't want to spend the evening in the bar." Yes, I said, I was game for another walk. I still had a lot of energy to work off. It was cool and inviting now outside. By starlight (there were no street lights then) we tried to retrace our afternoon's expedition. Outside the smaller houses we passed, we could see groups of people sitting by the light of tiny lamps, or even candles, and for a good deal of the way we saw nobody, although I was often conscious of the pad of bare feet nearby as we walked. We couldn't see where we were at all, and for all I knew we might have been walking in quite the wrong direction. Eventually we came out of the featureless dark and back to the Rest House.

My Rest House room was shared by another nursing sister, en route for Jos. She arrived while I was out. When I got back she was unpacking, and as I walked into the room she burst out laughing. "You aren't a bit like what I imagined!" she said – "I had expected a big buxom lady." It seemed that she had opened my wardrobe when looking to see which one was free for her, and she had noticed my shoes, which seemed to her to be very large. I explained that I had been advised to get shoes at least half a size larger than usual, in order to accommodate my feet which would swell with the heat.

9

Incidentally, talking about wardrobes, I was puzzled at first to find an electric light fitting inside the wardrobes in Lagos. I was told that all wardrobes were so equipped, and that one left the lights on at all times, because the climate there was so humid that unless you had that little bit of warmth (and therefore dryish air) everything went mildewed within hours. This was totally different from what I was to find in the Northern Region, where there was no humidity at all for three-quarters of the year.

About twenty-four hours later we were told that our train for Jos would leave the next morning, a Thursday. Our big loads, it seemed, had already gone, not to be seen again until we arrived at our respective postings. A Government agent took us to Lagos Railway Station. It seemed big and busy – most of the travellers being Africans, who, like the ship's deck passengers, took not only their personal luggage with them, but also all their food for the journey. Beggars abounded, moving with outstretched hands among the crowds waiting for trains. The whole place was seething with people and the noise was immense. There seemed to be no order, just chaos everywhere.

"Have you ever seen a tropical ulcer?" asked our escort, nodding towards a woman sitting by the barrier – another beggar – with a dirty bandage wrapped in a haphazard way round her leg, only half concealing the huge ulcer it was supposed to be covering. Nothing masked the stench coming from it. "You'll see – and smell – plenty of that," he added, as we passed the queues and were taken to our reserved compartment. First lesson in tropical medicine for me.

We settled in to our compartment – a sleeper in which the two bunks converted into a long comfortable seat for the daytime. There was also a tiny cubicle housing a minute washbasin and a loo. With a dining car not far away, we travelled luxuriously for the next forty-eight hours, looking with interest out of the window at the terrain through which we were passing. At first the surrounding country was thickly forested. Later on it gradually altered and the tall forbidding trees gave way to more open orchard bush and grassland. Occasionally I saw small settlements of mud houses, often enclosed with what looked like palisades made of branches or grass.

Now and again the train stopped – sometimes in the middle of nowhere for no apparent reason. We could be stationary for maybe up to an hour before starting off again. Once we stopped at Minna. There on the platform was a railway engine, mounted on a plinth. This was a museum piece of which Minna was very proud. It was the first railway engine ever to be used in Nigeria. An extraordinary thing to see in what seemed to be such a small place. We descended to the platform to have a bit of a walk up and down, a welcome change after all the hours of sitting still in the compartment. However, as white people we got so much attention from everyone else thronging the station that we returned to the train to escape it all. The platform was, as

I have indicated, packed with people – prospective passengers who, unless they were to travel first class, brought not only their personal luggage but also enough food for the length of time the journey would take. We, as government officers, always had first class travel provided – something I've rarely been able to do since, I may say.

The second night came, and we went to bed, leaving our suitcases to be 'finished off' in the morning, blissfully imagining that, Jos being the terminus, we would be allowed to sleep on until a respectable hour before being roused. Not a bit of it! We were woken at four thirty in the morning by the steward knocking frantically on our door, and shouting that we must get up immediately because "Dr Butler is waiting for you on the platform!" I remember sleepily thinking 'Who is Dr Butler?' before rolling out of my bunk, throwing on some clothes, casting the last few things pell-mell into my case, and leaving the train.

Dr Gordon Butler, it turned out, was the Senior Medical Officer (Jos). He bore us off to his house, to wait there until what he called a 'decent hour', when we could be taken to wherever we were to stay without getting anyone else up early to let us in.

I had, it seemed, been booked into Hill Station, a lovely country club-ish hotel, managed by one 'Pop' Bowler, who had run it for many years and who was a sort of legend in his own time. I should have been in the Government Rest House, but (luckily for me) it was fully booked, so Hill Station it was for me for the next few days until I was sent onwards to Maiduguri. We spent an enjoyable hour or so at Dr Butler's house, drinking tea and being well entertained by his pet chimpanzee, Charlotte. She liked to sit on one's knee and eat chocolate.

My time in Jos was really rather busy. First of all I was taken to buy a car. I think I put down some sort of deposit for it, but because a car was deemed to be necessary for one's work, Government operated an instalment system by which a set amount was deducted monthly from one's salary for two or three years. The whole process was quite painless. These finances had been so well worked out that generally by the time you had paid back the whole amount, your car had pretty well lived its life and you were just about ready to replace it. Cars didn't last as long out there as they do here in the UK. We reckoned in Nigeria that three years usually saw a car played out because of the nature of the roads which were mostly just sand. This invariably got into the works and gummed things up. Furthermore, when used regularly, the loose sandy surface wore down and you were left with lots of hard corrugations, and many potholes too. Did one drive slowly to take the corrugations easily and gently, but take an interminable time to cover the distances, or did one race along so that the corrugations were, so to speak, ironed out, and the journey made more quickly even though to do so juddered the car dreadfully? Whatever your decision, you still felt the constant vibration of the washboard-like surface as you went along it, and generally we all opted to go at speed because any journey usually involved long distances and journeys of several hours in any case, and nobody wanted to prolong travel times.

I chose an Opel estate car. I had been told by Dr Butler that British cars were not as suitable as foreign cars because they did not have such good ground clearance, which I'd need on the rough and sometimes rocky roads. I decided on an estate because I knew by then that I would be doing some touring and would need to pack camping kit, and also food and utensils, as well as personal luggage for me and for my cook, who would always come with me, and also for anyone else who needed to be taken with us.

In my letter home that week, I told my parents about my purchase, saying that I liked it very much. I commented that the insurance premium was 'enormous, due to the bad driving & high accident rate of Africans so that everyone has to pay the same – it will be about £58 per year!!!!' I added that luckily I would be given an allowance for my English no claim bonus. I also told them that the annual car tax was 'only £4.16', implying that it would have been more in England.

After an action packed sojourn in Jos, during which time I was also entertained well in the evenings by the medical department there, the day came when I booked out of Hill Station, got into my nice new car and set off for Maiduguri. This was the last stage of my long journey from England. I was told that the Government medical supplies lorry was going to Maiduguri at the same time, and that it would escort me so that help would be available in the event of any problems on the road. I was also told to make two overnight stops on the way, one at Bauchi and the other at Potiskum, this being so that I could get used to the nature of the roads which I would find tiring at first. Later I would do the whole hop in one day. The lorry led me out of Jos, and then dropped behind, for, said the driver, I would travel more quickly than he would, and if I had any difficulty I would know that he would eventually catch up and be able to help. I knew that I wasn't likely to get lost at any rate, the road to Maiduguri going straight there with barely a turning off it the whole way. I was looking forward now to the journey and my eventual arrival in Maiduguri. I was told that Dr Simpson, now going on leave, was to be replaced by Dr Louis Gonzalez, a fiery Irishman and a hard worker. I felt that this boded well. I liked hard workers and I liked to work hard myself.

I enjoyed my first day's driving, and in fact it wasn't a very long day for me, firstly because the road as far as Bauchi was tarmac-ed after a fashion.

12

It was also only a 90 mile stretch, scheduled so as to introduce me, as I said, gently to driving in Nigeria. I found that the roads were mostly not much more than one vehicle wide, even if tarmac-ed, so if by any chance you saw something coming, you simply drove off the road and into the edge of the bush alongside – which looked to me rather like a grass verge except that I realised it was only where trees had been hacked down roughly to make space for the road.

From time to time you would drive across a culvert – a sort of low bridge, under which in theory water would drain during the rains. The roads narrowed at culverts, where accidents could happen. People didn't seem to anticipate that somebody else might just be approaching a culvert at the same time as themselves; so head-on collisions could and did take place. One never caught up with or passed another car on the road, for motorcars travelled quickly, and were few and far between anyway. What we did try to pass were the lorries. They were never particularly fast, but were much more lumbering – and were often not in a very roadworthy state either. Because lorry drivers didn't ever seem to think that somebody might be waiting to pass, they didn't seem to use their wing mirrors at all – if in fact they had any. What they did instead was to have a boy or a young man riding on top of the loads behind the cab, whose job it was to keep a look out for traffic approaching from behind. In practice he too would not be watching all the time, and in fact was often to be seen lying down apparently asleep. However, should he see that somebody wished to pass, he would pick up a lump of wood – a bit of old plank, or a branch from a tree, or even as I once noticed, a stone – and he would toss it forwards over the top of the driver's cab. If the driver happened to notice that missiles were falling in front of his windscreen, he would pull over so that whoever was behind could get by. Often enough, as I say, you could safely bet that the lookout would not be looking backwards. I have travelled for miles behind these lorries, honking my horn almost non-stop before the boy suddenly heard me, or thought he had better look behind because he hadn't done so for some time. Once he started to throw his missiles forward, you had to be ready to shoot past quickly, while still trying to wait in case the driver had not noticed the wooden sticks being tossed over his head at first. The worst lorries to be stuck behind were those carrying dried fish. They smelt horrible!

Talking of roads and cars, I should say here that nearly all the cars had tubeless tyres. If one was punctured, it was a lot easier to deal with than one with an inner tube fitted, so we all carried tubeless tyre repair kits and foot pumps with us. It was not possible to buy tyres just anywhere, so we all had to try to be self-sufficient if we could. I was in the end a dab hand at jacking up my car and changing wheels – and mending punctures with rubber plugs.

On the early part of my journey I saw an occasional group of baboons, but they quickly vanished among the scrubby trees when they heard the car. The only other animals I saw on the whole of that journey were donkeys, goats, sheep and cattle. The donkeys were infuriating, for they seemed not to take any notice of cars or anything else. However, I forgave them to some extent because most of them were hobbled, having their forefeet tied together, so that they could not walk properly but had to progress by giving a sort of little hop with their front legs, only walking with their hind ones. Very difficult for them, but I suppose it was the only way in which they could be prevented from straying too far from their owners when not working. Poor little donkeys – they were all worked very hard, I thought – often carrying huge loads on their backs if they were not being ridden by men who sometimes looked as big as the animals themselves. They were never harnessed with saddles or reins when ridden – the rider simply sat on their backs, nearer to the hindquarters than the saddle area, and a stick was used to make them go. I think many of them had a tough time of it. I forgave them their apparent stupidity (maybe it was really stubbornness) because I felt they were so patient and hard working on the whole. Nevertheless, for car drivers they were a hazard, as were the other animals. Goats and sheep would walk along or across the road and never showed any inclination to move out of the way unless you were practically driving up their backsides! Likewise the cows that lumbered gently along. Actually the cattle were usually accompanied by a herdsman so that they would be hustled out of the way of traffic. But sometimes they wandered back into the road at just the wrong moment, with disastrous results to one's vehicle – not much difference from rural roads in the UK, then, except that cattle here will be more accustomed to passing traffic.

Bauchi behind me, I drove on the next day to Potiskum. Now the road was all laterite - no more tarmac. Laterite was reddish sand, which raised a lot of red dust -and underneath it all were the inevitable corrugations. Driving in deep sand was a bit like driving in deep soft snow, I thought. There were generally tyre tracks in it from the heavy lorries, and you found that you kept to these as much as you could. From time to time I would pass a few labourers with brooms who were smoothing the road surface as well as they could. They always waved and greeted anyone passing with lots of smiles. When I pointed ahead and asked "Potiskum?" I was answered with vigorous nods of the head and hands pointing onwards.

Finally, on 14th September, I set off on my last day's journey, feeling quite excited to think that in a few hours I would be in my own station. The road would be laterite for the remainder of the journey – and this was the longest lap. The car was soon covered with red sand as I was myself too - you had to have all the windows fully open all the time to get any feeling of coolness, so the sand and dust blew in and covered everything inside as well as out. Sunshine roofs were not usual then. The landscape rolled by, mile after mile, and the road passed through orchard bush, sometimes past large expanses of dry grassland, always with few signs of life. You could cover miles without seeing even a bird, and then maybe there would be one pedestrian, walking to who knows where. The sun beat down and took the colour out of the sky.

I was just starting to wonder how much further I had to go, when I saw, on my left, Maiduguri Airport. So far as I could make out as I drove along, it was just a tiny airstrip, but in spite of that I was to learn that it was classed as an international airport and an important point of departure for pilgrims for Mecca every year when the time for the Hadj came round. That was a busy time for the medical staff, as I will describe later. I knew now that I was pretty near to my station and my new life.

Three miles on, I found myself driving in the shade of tall leafy trees that bordered the road – neem trees, I found out. The shelter they gave from the blistering sun was such a relief, as was the look of the narrow green leaves. I was told that when Africa was opened up, seeds were brought and planted by people who had previously worked in India – neems were not actually native to Africa. Finally there was a cross roads and a signpost – 'To the Catering Rest House'. I followed the direction, along another road also shaded by trees, rising up a gentle slope for about another mile, finding myself eventually on the GRA (Government Reservation Area), where senior service officers, mostly at that time expatriates, were quartered. And there on a corner was the Rest House. I was more than ready to get out of the car for a good wash and a long cool drink.

I booked in and was allotted my chalet – bedroom, sitting-out verandah, bathroom. It felt like luxury after the road. While I was booking in, a lady came out of the dining room and greeted me warmly. "You're the new doctor," she said, "My name is Annie McGregor. You will come to our Scottish Country Dancing won't you? It's tonight!" Cautiously I said I wouldn't commit myself there and then, as I really wanted a little time to get my bearings, but I'd keep it in mind. In fact country dancing of any sort was never my scene, and at that particular moment the last thing I wanted to think about was jumping about in the heat trying to master an Eightsome Reel. But I thought she had been very kind and welcoming to me. My abiding memory of Annie McGregor whom I only met a very few times, as she moved away from the station not long afterwards, was of her vibrant personality and of her very warm welcome to me on my arrival in Maiduguri.

Having offloaded the car and got my belongings into the chalet, and having had a quick wash, I went back to the main rest house building, there to telephone Dr Simpson and tell him of my arrival. "I'll pick you up there straight after lunch," he said, "And I'll show you the hospital. You'll have to take it over tomorrow because I'm getting tomorrow's plane out and Dr Gonzalez, who should have arrived on the same plane when it comes in, has been delayed in Kano and won't be here for another week."

Chapter 3

I was totally taken aback at this – I knew absolutely nothing about local conditions, nothing about the general organisation of the hospital system, and had never done any hospital administration in the UK. Oh well, I thought, at least I could (I hoped) look after the patients.

Dr Simpson first took me to the house I had been allocated. It was locked up and would remain so until handed over to me officially by the Public Works Department. However, I was able to look in through the windows, protected, as were all windows in houses and Rest Houses then, with XPM. XPM? This was the abbreviation for Expanded Metal, which was a diamond shaped mesh that was fitted inside the windows as a guard against thieves. Thieves were still able to poke long poles through the spaces for the window handles, and thus hook any objects within reach, nevertheless. I wrote to my parents,

'I've seen the outside of my house – which is huge! But it looks a very beautiful one. The garden is just about big enough for a football ground!'

We went from there down to the hospital, driving back along the road to the GRA along which I had so recently driven to the Rest House. Instead of turning left towards the airport, we went straight on, and within yards were at the gateway to the hospital compound. It was cheek by jowl, I noticed, with one of the town's rubbish tips. When the Harmattan wind blew, it would send bits of paper and goodness knows what else in the way of trash, whirling into the grounds all round the wards. Not exactly ideal.

When we were just passing the turning off for the airport, I had noticed a small building with a sign on it. This announced that the building was 'Paddy Stokes' Memorial'. Who was Paddy Stokes, I wondered. It turned out that he was a previous Yard Superintendent for the Government Public Works Department (PWD), who had (hopefully) built this as a public toilet. I expect he had wanted to try to introduce some sort of public hygiene to the town. Alas, I never knew of its ever being used. A white elephant, but if nothing else, it was a talking point.

The hospital compound contained various wards – a male ward, a female ward, a children's ward, another for TB cases, and a small midwifery unit. The male and female wards held about 40 patients each. There were two further

17

buildings housing the outpatient clinics, one male, one female. There was another building which held the operating theatre, the X-ray Department, and a small office for the Matron, to which we would all repair halfway through the morning for a drink – coffee or warm squash (no refrigerator available there). I was to discover in the fullness of time that the X-ray Department was not always functional. Sometimes we had a radiographer, sometimes we didn't. Then, unless we had a go ourselves, no X-rays were available. Whether or not we had a radiographer made no difference if, as occasionally happened, a new stock of film was spoiled by the extreme heat of the climate as it was travelling to us from central stores hundreds of miles away – no X-rays could be taken anyway then.

There were three nursing sisters on the establishment – all expatriate. One was in charge and was the Matron. Another was Matron's deputy, and she also started off the female outpatient clinic each morning, sorting out patients she could treat herself and keeping back those who needed to see the doctor. And there was a third nursing sister – the 'Health Sister' who was, I suppose, a Health Visitor really. She didn't work within the hospital, but ran mother and baby clinics in the town and also did a great deal of bush touring, running similar clinics in outlying but not-too-far-away villages.

Another tiny building was grandly called the Pathology Laboratory, and was occupied by a technician who, with the aid of the few bottles of reagents which he had there, and one small microscope, looked at the various samples we sent over. Really there were not facilities for doing much more than checking for malaria, anaemia, parasites like hookworm and bilharzia and amoebic dysentery – and also testing for the ubiquitous venereal disease should this seem to be necessary. Usually the latter was only too obvious without further investigation.

We also had a small pharmacy, which sometimes had adequate supplies of medicines, but often it didn't. The pattern seemed to be that the pharmacist would always order far more than he really needed, hoping that something would arrive as a result, while the central stores always sent out much less than was requested. As a result, the pharmacist didn't throw anything away even if it had not been asked for by the time it passed its expiry date. If you did prescribe something a bit out of the ordinary, and it was 'expired', you had to make a judgement as to whether 'expired' meant simply that it was losing strength and therefore a rather larger dose than normal would still have some beneficial effect (reasoning that anything was better than nothing), or whether it would not be wise to give it at all, when you would have to manage without anything. A tight rein had to be kept on the supplies always, for it would have been so easy for someone to 'lose' a few medicines here and there. They could be sold very easily in the town at a profit – often diluted to make them go further. That was all another headache for the medical officers in charge. So much supervision had to be done in respect of every discipline because of the inherent corruption that went from top to bottom. I always thought it must have been hurtful to staff who were honest, though everyone, honest or not, knew how much dishonesty there was and that it had to be looked out for and stopped where possible. To try to prevent part at least of the illicit use of medicines, the Matron insisted that every empty penicillin bottle was checked, signed for and brought to her personally. She then had one of the hospital labourers smash every one (they were made of glass) with a hammer, right in front of her, so she knew that no bottle could be re-filled with water and then sold as penicillin in the town later on. What a carry on it always was, trying to keep tabs on medicines.

Behind the male outpatient clinic there were a few old buildings which had neither electricity nor running water, and which did not appear to be in use. I was to find out later what these were eventually used for.

Near the entrance to the hospital compound, and at a distance from the wards was another small building – normally kept locked. This was the mortuary. It contained a stone slab, a sink with one tap for running water (always assuming that the water was not cut off, which it often was); and a few instruments with which to perform autopsies. One didn't do very many of these because the Moslem population on the whole seemed to believe that death was part of life, and that as it was in any case, Allah's will, they were not happy at the idea of what they saw as unwarranted interference with the body after death. 'Causes of death' were not sought, although a post mortem would be agreed to if there was a legal requirement for it. For instance, I had to do one once when a man was brought in who had been murdered, so as to establish the actual cause of death for the court. The mortuary was hardly used otherwise, which was as well, because there was no refrigeration there, and in the hot climate...

However, Moslem practice meant that anyone who died should be buried before the sun set that day, or at the most within twenty four hours, so families usually took the dead away very quickly.

Finally, in the middle of the hospital compound, surrounded by everything else, stood the main administration block, with the doctor's office and that of the clerks. Neither room was very big, but they were enough for the work done there. The clerks' office contained various filing cabinets for records, and the medical officer's room contained a locked safe, which contained the DVA books and the petty cash. The senior clerk and the medical officer in charge each held a key for the safe – but both keys had to be used, each in a different lock, before the safe could be opened. What were DVA books? Yes, I wondered too, until I was told this meant 'Departmental Vote Account'.

This still didn't mean anything to me till it was explained that the 'vote' meant the allocation of money for all the different categories of things that were needed for both the hospital and for all bush dispensaries in the province. There would be one page for things like new theatre equipment; another for pharmacy stocks, and another for payment of locally employed people such as cooks, labourers and so on. The DVA books had to be kept under lock and key so that no false entries could be made in them, and the medical officer was personally responsible for all entries in them. It seemed a pity that if the money allocated for the year had not been spent because care had been taken with supplies, it could not be carried over for another year, but had to be returned to Government – i.e., the next year's allocation did not include anything left over from before. So as each year-end approached, the MO in charge would hasten to see what he might order that would benefit the hospital service, even if it was not yet needed. Sometimes this was allowed, sometimes not.

I discovered that the two medical officers (of whom I would now be one) between them were responsible not only for the hospital itself, but also for the satisfactory running of all the outlying Government dispensaries in the entire Province. This staffing and responsibility applied also to the Government hospital in Katsina, where I also worked later on. I learned that Bornu Province covered roughly 45,000 square miles – an enormous area.

The wards were an eye opener to me – different from anything I'd seen or imagined. They were like Nightingale wards, with beds along either side. Most of the beds did have mattresses and sheets on them. I thought the sheets looked rather dirty, and indeed some of them were, for patients who could get up would often use them to wrap round themselves, and they soon got grubby. However, we had a laundry and all sheets were washed when a bed was vacated. There were no washing machines – everything was done manually, and linen was hung on lines to dry, or spread on the ground. Luckily things dried in a matter of minutes except in the rainy season, and even then nothing took long, so drying was never a problem. Sunlight, I suppose, to some extent, burnt out the worst of any germs left on the bed linen, but if things were spread on the ground there was always the risk of Tumbu flies laying their eggs on them. The Tumbu larvae would burrow under one's skin and made abscesses, which could be a nuisance and rather nasty.

The ward floors were bare concrete, which gave the appearance of not being really clean, though they were washed and swept daily – swept more than once each day too. If all the beds were in use, and they almost always were, then extra patients were accommodated out on the verandahs in any spare beds available, and failing beds, on sleeping mats or mattresses

20

if available. These had to be put on the floor between beds. Relatives and friends would bring food in, though we did supply food for anyone without family. From time to time, relatives would also bring sleeping mats in and sleep there, so the place would be pretty crowded. On the children's ward, all the mothers stayed with their children, well, most of them tried to do so, so one would have to pick one's way between their sleeping mats and other impedimenta, though they did try to stow it all under the cots, sometimes even sleeping under the cots at night too. Except for the children's ward, one often had difficulty in distinguishing between real patients and their friends and relatives when a ward was particularly crowded. Although Dr Simpson tried to tell me the many diagnoses, I could not take very much in just then – there was so much and all of it new to me.

After the wards, he took me to his office and tried to explain to me the various administrative tasks I would have to take on for a week before his replacement, Dr Gonzalez, arrived. My mind was whirling by this time, and except for thinking that I was getting more and more bemused by it all, I was not much the wiser, and was just about to ask him to go over it again, more slowly, when a message came that a woman had been brought in with a bad miscarriage. The books were closed and bundled back into the safe and we were on our way to the maternity ward. Yes, she was certainly an emergency and had to be taken immediately into theatre.

"Will you give the anaesthetic?" said Dr Simpson, "While I get busy at the other end." I looked for the anaesthetic machine. Other than a cylinder of oxygen there was nothing that I recognised. Then the theatre nurse produced a metal facemask covered with gauze, and a bottle of chloroform. I hadn't given 'rag and bottle' anaesthetics since my early training days – anaesthetics had moved on a lot from there back in the UK. "It's the old rag and bottle," Dr Simpson told me. "We find that chloroform is the safest – there is some ether but as it is inflammable, we tend not to use it unless we have to, because of the climate. We have two or three ampoules of Pentothal, but we keep that for anything which simply cannot be induced by any other means as it is so scarce."

I was to discover that it was a red letter day if you had a spare doctor to give an anaesthetic – usually one of the theatre nurses gave it – chloroform too – and actually they were really surprisingly good. Only experienced nurses with some training did this generally, though the training in Africa at that time was not like what we had in England. However, some of the nurses had very little training, but had picked up – and had probably been shown – anaesthetic techniques from watching medical officers. This meant that the MO had not only to cope with operating alone with no other doctor to assist

21

(though you would have the senior theatre nurse to assist you) – but he or she also had to supervise the anaesthetic given by the nurse at the same time.

None of the theatre nursing staff, were expatriate, they were all African. Although very good and willing to do things correctly, I found that often they totally missed the point of some of the instructions we gave. For instance, the routine was that the instrument set should be boiled in the steriliser after use in theatre for twenty minutes before it could be used again. This meant, in my understanding, that nothing else should contaminate a set of tools while they were boiling up. However, I saw that if, for instance, an instrument slipped on to the floor, the nurse who was acting as theatre 'runner', picked it up and popped it immediately into the steriliser with the stuff already boiling there. This meant, of course, that nothing was really being boiled for its twenty minutes before a freshly contaminated item was added. So long as each thing had its time, in the eyes of the nurse, it didn't matter how often something new was added in. I never did manage to get this put right. I never saw any spinal anaesthetics used in all the years I was in Nigeria, though perhaps they were available in places like Kano or Lagos. Where I worked, we used locals for small ops where possible, and chloroform or ether for anything else.

Well, we finished in theatre, the patient was seen safely back into bed, and that seemed to be the end of what I was to do or be shown that day, though I would very much have liked to have an opportunity to go over it all again. Dr Simpson ran me back to the Rest House, simply saying on parting something on the lines of "Well, good luck, and can you pick us up in the morning and run us down to the airport? Louis will be here a week tomorrow, remember that you will have to meet his plane too". I spent that evening wondering how on earth I was going to cope, with such a rudimentary idea of how everything should be run. I hadn't even met any of the expatriate nursing sisters – did I even at that stage know that they weren't all on leave? Was there in fact any other expatriate or qualified person besides me working at the hospital? Oh well, I thought, at least I can look after the patients, and the books will just have to wait for a week.

Chapter 4

I did a very early morning ward round the next day and was back at the Rest House in time to collect Dr and Mrs Simpson and take them to the airport. I had, as I said, spotted it on my last run in to Maiduguri and had seen that it was only very small. Now I saw it from inside the perimeter, and it was indeed a tiny affair. It consisted only of a large flat area, cleared of all bush growth, along which there was just one runway – and not an enormously long one at that. Our local planes were fairly small, taking really only a handful of passengers. There was a small building containing, as I recall, just two rooms. One of these was the airport controller's office, and the other acted as a waiting area for passengers who wished to wait inside, and also as a storage area for any freight – of which there would never be very much other than the personal luggage carried by passengers. In fact the only freight I personally remember was my wedding cake – but that is a story to be told much later on in this memoir.

Our little planes did a regular circuit. We had two flights in and out each week. They connected up Lagos, Kano, Jos, Maiduguri and Yola. One flight would go one way round, and the other would do this in reverse. If one flight was fully booked, then you had to wait for the two or three days that would elapse before the next was due. This affected any onward passage to the UK for people going on leave – as did weather conditions too. In the event of tropical storms, planes could be – and often were, grounded or cancelled altogether. If your flight didn't happen, then you would have to wait for another three days before getting the next one, which could mean that any onward flight from Kano, whether an internal flight or an international one, would be delayed too, for anything between several hours to several days. Such was the transport system in those days.

Back to Maiduguri airport. Aeroplane day was quite an event in Maiduguri, and anyone who could be spared would go down to see the plane come in. It was a little outing for us to go there, almost a social occasion. It was fun seeing who was going on leave, and who was arriving back. You could give last minute messages for your families to those going on leave – once arrived in London, they would telephone one's family, who would feel they had real up to date information as to how you were and what you were doing. It was nice to know that there was such a connection every so often. Letters didn't take all that long – only a few days or a week, but a personal message, delivered by someone who might have seen you the day before was exciting for families. There was no international phone connection possible for us then – not from Maiduguri, anyway. And of course, mobile phones did not exist then.

The airport was a good place to go to for a walk with children too. There was never any danger of accidents, and they could run about happily with a ball. It was a change for them from one's own compound and we did try to give them different things to see and do. When you had very young children, still buggy-bound, it was much easier to wheel the buggy along the runway, which was covered with tarmac and therefore smooth, as compared with trying to drag it through the deep soft sand of the roads on the GRA.

The Simpsons and I chatted for a while, and then the little plane swooped down for its landing and rolled to a halt. The passengers began to disembark. To the Simpson's surprise and to my great relief, one of the arrivals was Dr Louis Gonzalez, coming into Maiduguri on time after all. It turned out that, having problems over getting a new car, he had first telegraphed that he would be delayed. Then later on, when things slowly began to resolve over his car, he telegraphed again to say that he would arrive after all as originally planned, but would have to go back to Kano a week later to pick up the new car and bring it back. His telegrams had arrived in the reverse order. But that was Nigeria – lots of things happened like that. Anyway, I was never so glad to see anyone in my life.

Louis was a great chap to work with. He was, as I had been told, quite a fiery man, but also infinitely kind and compassionate, though he did not suffer fools gladly. He worked tremendously hard and did not spare himself. He was well liked by everybody who knew him, and deservedly so. A life long bachelor, Louis was a devout Catholic. I remember that he never ever operated, all the time I worked with him, without first crossing himself and offering up a brief prayer that everything would go all right for his patient, before he made the first incision. He ran his household on oiled wheels and took pride in having things like Waterford glass and good silverware on his table. "I've been out here for many years," he would say, "and while I'm here, this is my home. I see no reason not to have it as comfortable and as nicely appointed as if I lived back in Ireland." Quite right too, he was. He was also passionately fond of classical music, especially, I recall, of grand opera. He had a gramophone and many records, saying that, when his music was on he would shut all his windows so that he could 'conduct' the orchestra and sing along with his operatic music without disturbing anyone else. Louis remained a friend of ours from my first meeting him until his death many years later, long after we had all retired from Nigeria.

So here I was on the second day in my station, mightily relieved to know that somebody was here with me who knew the ropes, and that although he was to return to Kano a week later, it would only be for forty eight hours. I was confident that I would cope for that short time. Meanwhile I still had to move into my house.

As I said earlier, from the outside it looked huge to me – and indeed the rooms were all a good size – much bigger than in our house in England. There was a large central lounge from which, through an archway, one walked into a smaller dining room. A door from that opened into a sort of butler's pantry (for lack of a better description). That had a sink in it with a tap, but no cooking stove. A lockable storeroom opened off this. The only other door there was the back door into the compound, and a yard or two away was the cook's kitchen – a small building, separate from the rest of the house. Here all meals were prepared. The cooking was all done on a wood burning stove, with hot plates for pans on top and an oven at the side. I discovered that I would have to buy a cord of wood and hire a man to chop it up into serviceable chunks.

From the lounge on the other side was a door leading to a short corridor, off which on one side was a spare bedroom, while opposite that another two doors opened into the bathroom and loo respectively. At the end of the corridor a door opened into the main bedroom, which was enormous. At the far end of this in turn were double glass doors opening on to a small outside area surrounded by a tall hedge of a flowering shrub, Pride of Barbados. This was, I found out, my 'sleeping out area'. Everyone, I was told, slept outside in the hot season. The hedge continued right round the front of the house. It was very decorative, with red and yellowish flowers – but had to be pruned regularly because it grew so quickly. It was pretty, though.

The dining room, lounge and main bedroom all had ceiling fans, which were a help in the climate, but any guest would have to make do with just a table fan – also provided in the lounge, but which I took into my bedroom (the main one) and had by my bedside whirring away right through the night as well as having the ceiling fan switched on. Even so, my sheets and nightwear would be damp with sweat in the mornings.

Throughout the house were innumerable windows, for all of which I had to make curtains. Having been told by Mrs Simpson before I left England how many yards of material I would need, I had taken advantage of the summer sales to stock up on curtaining as well as other household goods. Now I had to get busy with the sewing, using the tiny sewing machine that I had brought with me. It turned out to have been an invaluable purchase, and with it I made up curtains for all the houses I lived in, as well as innumerable cotton dresses, blouses, skirts, underwear, and later on my children's clothes, through all the years I was out in Nigeria. It was one of my most prized possessions, as was also the miniature camp cooker I had taken out with me. I continued to use both of these from time to time after we retired from the service and lived permanently in the UK, until they inevitably gave up the ghost through so much wear and tear.

My first week in Maiduguri was totally taken up with the hospital and curtain making in any spare moments, but at last I was able to relax and draw breath. I was also plunged into a whirl of social and official activities, the like of which I had never experienced before. When anyone new came into a station, they were immediately invited round for drinks or dinner or Sunday curry lunches by everyone else. Partly this was in order to make the newcomer welcome and able to meet as many people as possible quickly – and partly because, especially in a small station, a new face meant news from outside, and a fresh angle on conversation and ideas.

The expatriates between them represented a wide cross section of professional skills, and we worked in many different departments. There were people working in the Education Department, any of whom could be posted at any time to take on very different tasks – from administrative duties to teaching in Government schools, or lecturing in colleges. There was my own department, the Medical one, with the doctors and senior nursing staff. Other government officers worked in the Forestry Department, the Posts and Telegraphs Dept., the Audit Department and the Geology Dept. We had Veterinary Surgeons and we had the Provincial Engineer in charge of the civil engineering in a province. There were the Irrigation people (affectionately known to us all as the 'well-diggers'), who lived and worked very often for weeks on end out in the bush, coming into station only occasionally for a few days to stock up on supplies and live it up for a bit amongst our few 'bright lights' before returning to camp life and tough work. There was the Yard Superintendent, who oversaw the Public Works Department, and several expatriate staff working with him. There were people of all nationalities who looked after the various commercial firms, John Holt's, Chellaram's, CFAO (a French company), Leventis (Greek), UAC (United Africa Company), so we met and socialised with French, Greek, Lebanese, and Indian personnel in addition to the British expatriates. Within the Medical department itself, from time to time we had doctors from other countries too, and in my time I worked with medical officers from India, Egypt, Saudi Arabia, Malaysia, and Germany as well as with one of the first graduates from the first Nigerian medical school. The Education department also took teaching staff from other countries, and one rubbed shoulders with Americans, Australians and New Zealanders as well as officers from the Indian subcontinent. My impression from across the years is that the international aspect of

Government staffing was more pronounced after Independence. Then there were expatriate officers working in the banks – Barclay's Bank DCO, and the British Bank of West Africa (BBWA). And finally (I don't think I've missed anyone out) there were the Superintendents and Assistant Superintendents of the Nigeria Police.

In Kaduna, the administrative headquarters of the Northern Region, there was also a legal department, whose staff visited us lesser mortals from time to time (as did senior personnel from other departments). It was really a very interesting mix, and I found it fascinating to be able to meet people from so many areas of work very different from my own.

Other than the one small cinema in the town, and the annual Agricultural Show and occasional race meetings, we had to make our own entertainment. There were other stations where there was nothing at all except what you could provide in the way of entertainment in your own houses, so we were actually quite lucky in Maiduguri. However, we all tried very hard to do what we could to have each other in for meals and to lay on a good evening. Generally one entertained at weekends, for most of us were pretty tired by the end of the day during the week.

We all worked hard, and the working day started pretty early. Medical staff and education staff were always on call – the Government education establishments were all boarding institutions – but most other people were free after the working day finished around 2 p.m. The usual pattern was to get one's head down after lunch for a siesta, because the heat was so great. Then, at about 4 o'clock, people began to surface. Some would go to the Club, perhaps to get books from its library, or to play snooker or table tennis, or simply to socialise. In some stations there were proper tennis courts – and even, though rarely, a 'golf course' but nothing like we see here in the UK. Others of us did a bit of riding once the day became cooler – you could usually manage an hour before darkness fell – and all of us were happy to call on friends or to have people call on us, and then we all sat on our verandahs clutching the inevitable long cold drinks and talking. In Maiduguri the Senior Service Club also boasted a small swimming pool, though after it had been emptied, cleaned and refilled you had to wait for a day or two before swimming because the water it had been filled with was too hot – the water was from storage tanks, which were heated by the sun all day long. The pool only cooled down after enough evaporation had happened.

There were other ways in which we entertained ourselves too. Sometimes play-reading groups were established. Occasionally, depending upon what talent there was in a station, plays (or pantomimes at Christmas) were actually performed. These went down very well, as might be imagined. And there was always, as indicated by my first greeting in Maiduguri, Scottish Country Dancing for anyone energetic enough at the end of the day to take part.

Everyone took trouble over dinner parties. Women put on their prettiest dresses and the men wore 'tropical' weight light suits and ties – though they were always invited to discard their jackets after arriving, and would do so. Dinners were rather formal – not because we were all fuddy-duddy beings, but because to be formal signalled some relief from the day's extreme heat and stickiness, and because therefore one felt more like eating food, and because it made a change and was good for us to take trouble over things. It was fun to dress up a bit and for once to be able to wear a little lipstick without it melting. Lipstick, if you used it at all, had to be kept in the fridge, by the way, otherwise it became soft and practically liquid within minutes. I soon threw out all my other make-up because it simply ran off my face in the heat.

One of my early invitations was for dinner at the Residency. When you first went to a station, one of your initial duties was to go and sign the 'Resident's Book.' In Maiduguri this was kept on a table in a large grass hut at the gateway to the Residency. The gateway always had a Native Authority policeman on duty there. He would take you inside and there would be the book, already open at the right page. This custom was necessary because the Resident needed to know who was in station officially. He would also need to be told if anyone was posted away or going on leave. The Resident was the Government representative, and was responsible for his province. He had to know what was going on everywhere and he conducted the provincial administration.

Once Federal Independence was established, the Residents' appointments came to an end, and Nigerian Provincial Commissioners were appointed instead. But for the time being, the British Resident was the 'father' of the province. Not only did he work in the provincial headquarters, but he also regularly toured the province to make sure that he knew it all, and was seen by the inhabitants, who regarded him always with great respect and knew that they could bring problems to him which would be sorted out. Nigeria was governed through 'Indirect rule' which meant that the Emirs and their Native Authorities had their own administration in their own areas, but this was, to put it simply, overseen by the British administrators with a light but firm touch as and when necessary. The two administrations worked together extremely well, as far as I could see. Residents were also, needless to say, responsible for the general demeanour of the expatriates on their 'patch'. If anyone overstepped the mark, the Resident would send for him (or her) to sort out the situation. If necessary, and in an extreme case, an expatriate could be dismissed from post and sent home.

An invitation to the Residency was a bit like a royal command. You did not refuse unless you had to be out of station and therefore unable to accept. Everyone sooner or later would be invited there, and if you were new then to invite you for dinner was an opportunity for the Resident to meet you in a very nice way. If the Resident (with or without wife) was at any other event to which you were also present, the convention was that nobody left before they did, unless there was a very good reason, for instance, if one of the medical officers was called to the hospital. And here I should note that as almost nobody had telephones except the MOs and the Principals of the Government Educational establishments, the doctors certainly could not accept invitations out if they were on call, unless they lived very near to where they were invited. In such case, one's houseboy, if he was familiar with a telephone, could answer and run round with a message to where one was. Telephones, by the way, operated via wet batteries that looked like the old accumulators used for wireless sets many years ago. If the phone didn't work well, you topped up the battery with water, for things evaporated fast in the climate.

Another official visit, equivalent to the signing of the Resident's book, was that of going to see and be received by, the local Emir, or, in Maiduguri, the Shehu of Bornu. Accordingly, Louis and I, having been so summoned, were conducted by the Native Authority Health Representative to the Shehu's palace. This was a large building, which at first glance looked to me to be almost modern in style, but which, when you got inside, was clearly not as new as it appeared to be. It was at the end of a wide road, the Dandal Way, which seemed almost as wide and long as a military parade ground. It was here that local durbars were held, with the horsemen processing down the whole length of it, with a mad gallop for the final few yards. I shall talk about the durbars later on, suffice it to say here that they were exciting and impressive.

We were taken inside the palace to the Shehu's reception room. This was also quite large and rather dark – I wasn't conscious of windows though there must have been some. At the far end of it was a sort of dais, piled with cushions, and there sat the Shehu. He was a very old man, rather frail, though he took part in as many official occasions as he could still – notably tapping in the first stake signifying the beginning of the building of a railway to Maiduguri. The stake was where the station would be built.

Louis and I stood near the door to the reception hall, while the Shehu was seated yards away from us, as I said. He was attended by several people, all in colourful robes. Some were simply seated by his side, others, servants no doubt, were fanning him slowly with huge feather fans. All seemed to hold him in great respect. The rich colours of the clothes they all wore, and the brightly dyed ostrich feathers of the fans, the exotic dark and almost mysterious surroundings made me think of all the Tales of the Arabian Nights I had read.

Our escort spoke to him in Kanuri (although I think the Shehu actually did speak a few words of English, he preferred on occasions such as these to use his own language). He was told who we were, and we were introduced to him by name, one by one. The Shehu then made his acknowledgement through an interpreter, welcoming us to Bornu, and wishing us a happy and successful tour. After a moment or two, during which he asked a few rather formal questions – where had we come from, did we enjoy being in Nigeria and Bornu, that sort of thing, we were ushered out, the duty done. I saw the Shehu on several other occasions, mostly official ones when I was merely part of a huge gathering of people – durbars, the railway 'opening', occasions of visits of important visitors such as the celebration of Federal Independence, when Princess Alexandra came to Bornu.

I was also, at about that time, introduced to the Waziri of Bornu – Shettima Kashim Ibrahim, who was later to become the Governor of Northern Nigeria and to be knighted. He was, as I was to realise over the months, a very nice man indeed. Tall, with great dignity and wisdom, coupled with a dry sense of humour, he dealt with all the local administration in the name of the Shehu. When I married, he was kind enough to send us a wedding gift, though was unable to attend the wedding itself. At the time I first met him, I had told my parents that I thought he was a 'kind of Minister (of State)' and I suppose I'd pretty well got the idea. We all respected him, Europeans and Africans alike.

Chapter 5

Things happened so quickly in my first week or two in Maiduguri that I hardly know where to start. My weekly letters home to my parents reflect the kaleidoscope of impressions that whirled round me at this time. My father died some thirty years before my mother, and it was only all those years later, when I cleared the house, that I discovered he had kept almost all of my letters from the moment I left England until the week before he died. They were tucked away at the back of a cupboard in the garage, with his tools. It was a most moving moment to me, and at the same time, fascinating to read my initial impressions on arriving in Nigeria, and to see again how I coped with such a different way of life and culture. I experienced once more my culture shock and my reactions as I adapted to everything and learnt to love the places I lived in and the people amongst whom I worked.

Once in my house, I see that I had felt so menaced by what everyone had told me about thieves that for some time I kept my bedroom windows closed at night, thus sweltering where I might have felt a bit cooler. Similarly I slept very badly for my first night or two there, being disturbed by what I gradually realised were quite normal 'house noises', but which I imagined at first to be the noises of somebody trying to break in. In fact we were only burgled once during all the years in Nigeria.

I engaged two house-boys. The more senior was Samuel, my cook-steward, who came with a good reference from another expatriate; and Amadu who came as my 'small boy', or junior steward. He had worked for Dr and Mrs Simpson, and was still learning his job. He was in fact a fairly young lad, a teenager. He was a good little lad, tried hard and I liked him. His only fault was to have large groups of his friends up to the house where they all sat with him round my back door. I felt that he should see his pals in his own quarters (all house staff had quarters provided for them within your compound), and not by my open door, where it would be very tempting for one or two of them to go into the house and have a good look round to see if there was anything worth taking. Mrs Simpson had warned me that Amadu did seem to have all his friends up in this way, but said she just reminded him now and again, and it was all kept under control. Looking back, I think I was probably rather hard on both Samuel and Amadu to start with – and I think they were both very patient with me when I was still so clearly new and feeling my way. But we all settled down and they looked after me very well, anticipating jobs often before I drew things to their attention.

31

Some people I met, who were very kind to me and had me round to their house for meals, kept two dogs – a sort of cross between red setters and spaniels. The female had just had pups, and I was promised one if I wanted, when it was old enough. I looked forward to this, thinking that the pup would be a good companion (he was) and also perhaps a good guard dog later on (he was that too).

My days settled into a routine. At quarter to six each morning I got up, bathed and dressed. The bath water was always lovely and cool then because I filled up the bath last thing at night so that evaporation would cool it down. Then, half an hour later, I unlocked the doors and let the boys in. Within minutes Samuel had brought me a pot of tea and at a quarter to seven I went off to the hospital, where I would try to do a quick ward round before going into the male outpatient clinic. Two or three times a week, however, we operated, and on those days we went in to theatre first thing, so as to get as much as possible done there while it was still relatively cool. Even so, we were usually wringing wet by the time we came out. We did have a ceiling fan in theatre, just above the operating table, but there was nothing like air conditioning available for us. What with the effect of having to wear heavy rubber aprons as well as gowns, masks and rubber gloves, it was really pretty hot while we worked. Many theatre facilities that we took for granted in the UK were not available to us in Maiduguri. We had, for instance, no diathermy. Although I had qualified before diathermy came to my unit at Manchester Royal Infirmary, it had arrived there a couple of months later on, and to be without it so many years later felt strange. We had no electrical suction apparatus either, which meant that it took longer to keep a clear operating area. Anyway, what was the use of electrical equipment in a place where the electricity supply could be cut off from time to time? Better to carry on with the older ways and be sure that you could cope even if it took longer.

We tackled all sorts of conditions in theatre, because there was nobody else to operate but us. Chiefly our surgical work seemed to consist of things like hernias, amputations and gynaecological work of all kinds. And there were always trauma cases from every imaginable cause. From time to time there would be a Caesarean section or the removal of retained products of conception either from a miscarriage or from a birth where the whole placenta had not come away entirely. We also found that a surprising number of women in and around Maiduguri had enormous and multiple fibroids and a great deal of our surgical work for women was the removal of these. Occasionally we could remove them altogether, but often there were so many, that we had to remove the whole uterus in order to give the poor women any relief from their symptoms. The usual comment when these women came into the outpatient clinic was "I have been pregnant for two years, or fourteen months, (or however long they had had symptoms) – but yet no baby". The problem was that these tumours were often so many that they bulked up the womb to the size of a full term pregnancy, or sometimes even larger than that. No wonder the women asked us why they had not yet gone into labour. These fibroids must have been very heavy and wearying to carry about, and of course people could get anaemic because of them too.

In addition to all the above problems, I found myself doing various orthopaedic operations. Louis was not keen on orthopaedics, whereas I had learnt a lot from my time at Beverley, where as well as being primarily the Resident Medical Officer, I had also acted as houseman to the orthopaedic surgeon there. I was always grateful for what he had taught me. Louis told me to "set up my own little corner of orthopaedics" in both male and female wards, and he very happily let me take over all the orthopaedic work from then on. I enjoyed it, and I like to think that the nursing staff on the wards learnt a bit from me in turn, because I managed, by rummaging round in several store cupboards, to unearth all sort of splints and tractions which they had never seen used. The main problem, where there were open fractures, was that of infection. The hot climate meant that bugs could – and did – multiply very fast, and as so many people were rather debilitated because of things like malaria, or hookworm and so on, they succumbed easily to infections. It was not always easy to save limbs, and many amputations that might have been avoided in a more temperate climate, had to be done because of severe infections, apart from any accompanying debilitation from other causes. I remember a patient who came in with multiple fractures of his leg – open ones – because he had been bitten by a crocodile. Hopefully I set up a system of tractions for him, together with intensive antibiotic treatment. In theory we should have won out, but in fact, the infection took over within a very short time, and I had to take his leg off. The people who brought him into hospital (he had travelled about a hundred miles to get to us) told me that he was a 'very good crocodile caller – he calls them and they come out of the water to him'. This time, they had come a bit too near! Perhaps the animals had become tired of having to go to him every time he called them up.

Other problems resulted from the practice of plastering up wounds with a mixture of dung and sand. No doubt we would not see the outcome of this treatment in many instances when people did not attend the hospital, and no doubt many would heal up well in spite of their dressings. What came to us were wounds which did not heal, perhaps because they were too severe anyway and needed more specialised treatment, but more often because they became infected. I was surprised too, to see that a common treatment among

33

the locals for pain in any part of the body was either to brand it with a hot iron, or alternatively to 'cup' it with the end of a cow's horn which had been heated – a blistering treatment. This was really a quite medieval attempt to use what we now call 'counter-irritation' – that is, the production of a different pain which masked the first one.

So much of what I saw in Nigeria took me back through history and I am not writing of simply medical things now. Just going about the town one constantly saw scenes looking just like the pictures in books back in the UK of times long gone – men in long flowing robes, some wearing turbans; women similarly in long gowns and head coverings, people riding patient little donkeys, others on horseback, yet others on camels, leading long caravans in from the desert. Where western garments and technology had developed and altered over the centuries, here things seemed to be timeless and unchanging. In a letter to my family I wrote,

'26.2.1958

There was such a contrast in ancient and modern. The other day I was passing the place where they are drilling for water, with all sorts of erections like a great meccano set up in the air and machinery of all kinds scattered about, and also watching it were the drivers of a long string of camels coming from the market. The camels were standing looking most frightfully superior, as only camels can, and not taking the slightest notice of the goings on around them, as if to say, "We got along just as well in Biblical times as we do now, what's all the fuss about?" '

One could imagine them adding, with a scornful sniff, "We shall still be here, plodding along, doing what we have always done, when you are long gone to be replaced with something else."

At nine o'clock it was officially breakfast time, and everyone went home for half an hour, maybe for the luxury of a whole hour. If we were in theatre we hoped to finish in time for that, but otherwise went when we could, or missed breakfast out that day. Never a big eater, I only ever had a plate of fresh fruit salad and more cups of tea then (my cooks must have thought I was very boring, never wanting even any toast and certainly not a cooked meal). The fruit was very refreshing and always went down well. If I had been up in the night, I would try to have ten minutes or so on my bed – even perhaps snatching a few minutes of sleep, as every little helped, before getting back to work.

In Maiduguri there was a small nursing home on the GRA. It had first been set up in World War Two by the Americans to serve as a small hospital for men who were posted out there. Many years later I met a doctor back here in the UK who had been in the British Forces and who had been in Maiduguri during the war. He remembered the nursing home there as being the forces' hospital. Now it was for Government Senior Service personnel. However, when I first went there, we hadn't got enough nurses to staff it full time, so it was only opened for half an hour two or three times a week for outpatient surgeries. Some years later we were able to staff it and open it permanently, and in fact my second child was born there, although at the time I am writing about – my first months in Maiduguri – I had not yet met the man I was to marry. Usually there were not many patients to be seen, and if there was any emergency, people knew that they could always call on Louis and me for help anyway. But one of us had to attend regularly if for nothing more than to do the mandatory medicals for expatriate officers before they went on leave.

If any expatriate or other senior officer needed hospital treatment, then unless we could manage to find staff for the time needed, patients had to be sent to Kano for admission to Nassarawa Hospital there. Luckily, during my time, we only had to send one person onwards and he was so ill that I had to accompany him on the local plane for that journey. This meant that I had a few days at a loose end in Kano until the next plane back to Maiduguri was available. Louis was left to hold the fort on his own, while I lived it up for forty-eight hours in Kano, which in fact gave me an opportunity to do a little shopping for items that were unobtainable in Maiduguri.

If it was not a nursing home day, then after breakfast I would get straight back to the main hospital in town and carry on with the outpatient clinic. On days when we did not operate first thing, I would have started outpatients at 7 o'clock, so that with luck I would have cracked the bulk of the male clinic by 9 o'clock, and hopefully would only have to 'mop up' before going across the compound to the women's clinic. These clinics were nothing like those in Britain.

From an early hour people would be arriving. The male clinic had a large indoor area where they could wait, but even so, the ever increasing number of people wishing to be seen would overflow out into the compound, and to get inside I would have to pick my way among a crowd of men and boys sitting in the sand waiting. Inside, one of our male nurses would have started working, and he tried to weed out patients with whom he could deal himself – dressings, for instance, for abrasions, or for the great tropical ulcers which abounded. I would only see the worst of these because there were so many. Ailments varied from the minor to more serious ones. A common complaint

– one that a great proportion of patients had was, "Doctor, I have fever and pains all over." The most likely diagnosis was that of malaria. I always sent them to the lab for a blood test, to confirm this – and appropriate treatment would be started immediately, before I had the result – but in any case, most people would harbour the parasites, as malaria was endemic. Treatment could only help even if there was something else to be found as well. Most of these cases were well again in a couple of days, as the general population had some degree of herd immunity – that is, although they had the parasites and did get symptoms from time to time, they had developed over the generations some ability to battle malaria and cope with it. However, treatment helped in the case of exacerbations – or seemed to do so.

Of course people had other things that caused 'fever and pains all over' – and these had to be investigated too. Many patients suffered from bilharzia – due to a parasitic infection carried in running water. They would notice that there was blood in their urine, and that brought them to the hospital. The treatment consisted of a long course of injections. Sadly, the relapse rate was high because people still had to live in the same conditions as they always had, and few heeded the advice to store water in containers so that it became stagnant and therefore free of the parasite. In any case, water was a precious commodity for many, and their only source would be a local stream, if there was one – or they would have to buy water from a local water carrier, and where did he get it from? There were also wells – but these would not always be clean. Early in the day there would almost always be a group of women by the wells, collecting their water for the day. Even if the well was a 'clean' one, you would notice many of the women sweeping their hand across the water surface if it was near enough to reach – so as to push aside any debris or weed that was there before they dipped their containers in – a habit long ingrained from the days when artesian wells had not been dug – and probably still necessary in outlying places anyway.

In some places there were standpipes with taps, where the water was probably OK.

There was actually a great deal of water available underground – and any regular supply which did come through taps was from artesian wells, but few people in the towns and villages had a supply from taps as we did in Government accommodation. Even so, we did not drink it as it came out of the taps. Every Government house was supplied with a water filter. You boiled all water for drinking and tooth cleaning, and then poured it into the filter container, where it had to seep through the filter cartridge into the lower half from where you turned a small tap and got your drinking water. You had to acquire as many empty glass bottles as you could, because the water was poured into them from the filter, and they were put into the fridge to cool – you couldn't drink boiling hot water! It wasn't hard to get bottles because you went through so many bottles of squash all the time in an effort to keep properly hydrated, there were always plenty about the place.

Malaria and bilharzia were only two of a myriad syndromes we saw. There were cases of pneumonia, especially during the rainy season when it could be cooler at times as well as wet. There were eye problems of all sorts as well as intestinal syndromes from simple cases of the 'runs' to amoebic dysentery. There were skin problems of all kinds, and there were infectious diseases too. Many children had measles, and in passing I note that African measles seemed to be much more severe than the British variety, even in children who were not debilitated beforehand. To point this up, my own children caught measles from an English boy whose parents had just returned from leave – he developed measles about a couple of days after their arrival. My two certainly had measles but were no more ill than I would have expected. A year or two later however, an African child with whose parents we were friendly, came to our house with her mother and played briefly with my two. Her mother contacted us a day or so later to say that the little girl had got measles. I hoped mine, having had it already, would escape a second attack. But no, they both went down with measles again, were quite ill this time and in fact my daughter was so very ill that I thought we were going to lose her.

Another illness that we would have to deal with from time to time was rabies. Occasionally somebody would have been bitten by a rabid animal – generally a dog, and would be brought to the hospital for treatment. If they were brought immediately then we would give a course of anti-rabies injections, after which, hopefully, the patient would not be affected. However, at times we had somebody who had developed the disease, and it was horrible knowing that there was absolutely nothing that we could offer, apart from careful nursing and sedation. At such times our prime responsibility was to the staff who cared for the patients. We all had to undergo the full course of anti-rabies shots straight away. Patients suffering from rabies, especially if they became delirious, could and did become aggressive, spitting, biting and scratching those who looked after them, and this could transmit the infection to others. I well remember a child who had rabies and who, in her disorientated condition, bit or spat at anyone who came near to her, and resisted all attempts to wash her or make her bed. We all started our injections at the same time. The injection was quite a large one – and you had to have a shot each day for, I seem to remember, ten or fourteen days. I used to give my own each evening when I bathed and changed out of my workaday clothes. Not a treatment one would choose to have just for fun, but infinitely preferable to having the disease.

People were, understandably, terrified of rabies. I must say that it was the one thing that I viewed with great respect, knowing that once established, nothing could be done for it. Every dog that bit was described by its victim as 'mad' whether it was or not, and obviously, until proved otherwise we had to accept peoples' statements. Anyone who had been bitten was asked to catch the animal concerned, if at all possible, and take it to the Veterinary Department. If the vet found that any animal in the station was indeed rabid, he would immediately issue a 'rabies order'. This meant that all pets had to be confined to the house, tied up there if necessary, until enough time had passed to make sure things were safe again. I was always watching my young dog for untoward symptoms, particularly as at one time he took to joining a pack of bush dogs for some of their jaunts. Luckily he (having had his anti-rabies shots previously) was always OK, but still had to endure being confined to the house during a rabies order. He hated this, needless to say. Other dreaded diseases, Lassa fever, Marburg disease, Ebola fever, and AIDS, were not known about in those days, so that rabies was the worst thing we could think of.

I was surprised at first, though why I should have been I don't really know, to find that I was seeing many diseases, like pneumonia, measles, mumps and so on, that I saw in England, as well as lots of tropical diseases. I think I had expected everything to be tropical. Familiar things I could deal with easily, but I had a lot of reading to do for the others at first.

As usual, I am digressing. Back, then, to outpatients at the main hospital. Generally, as I said, the nursing staff would deal with what they could out of the press of patients, but all the rest had to be brought through to the medical officer. As one could see anything up to a hundred people in one clinic, though fortunately not quite so many as a general rule, one could not give very much time to each. Moreover, quite a lot of time was taken up with all the interpreting that had to go on. There were about four languages which were spoken much of the time – Hausa, Kanuri, Fulani, and Arabic. Until I learnt a bit of Hausa, everything had to be translated for me.

I was always amazed at how much venereal disease there was among both men and women, though one was more aware of it in the men because their symptoms were usually more overt. The male nurses were more than abrupt with these patients – partly, I suppose, because there were simply so many of them, and partly because the quality of kindness and/or gentleness as I understood it, was missing here. Life was tough out here, and especially in outlying areas, help not easy to obtain. People suffered all sorts without complaining. The thing was to survive. If you didn't, then hard luck. It was the way things were.

Anyway, I would be presented with man after man suffering from gonorrhoea. One by one they would be brought in front of me. "*Menene?*" I would ask – 'What is your trouble?' "*Ciwon Sanyi*" would be the reply 'White trouble' or 'White water coming'. "Show the doctor your prick!" the nurse would command, and there would be the unmistakeable evidence. I wonder how many gallons of penicillin we dispensed over the years, and I wonder what difference has been made over the years. Very little, I would imagine, if the AIDS epidemic is anything to go by. Incidentally, the ladies of the night in Maiduguri were not spoken of as 'prostitutes', but as 'harlots'. I never heard any African use the word 'prostitute'.

I was appalled at the amount of venereal disease I saw at first. But one got used to it being just a fact of life there. I did manage, I hope, to do my bit in battling against it several years later when I set up a local school medical service, and gave talks to some of the older pupils/students at the schools and colleges. The first classes I spoke to seemed to have taken what I told them on board, but I wonder if the message carried on. I shall never know.

After dealing with the male outpatients, I would have to cross the hospital compound and see what was waiting for me in the female clinic. One of the expatriate nursing sisters – the deputy matron – would have dealt with what she could while I was in the male outpatient clinic, and I would catch up with what she had left for me. There were never quite as many women waiting as there were men – perhaps because women could not leave the households and families as easily – perhaps they were not allowed to by their husbands, who knows? Some seemed to have quite a bit of independence and came and went as they pleased, but many did not.

Again there were many and varied problems, including a great deal of gynaecological trouble. Due to poor midwifery out in the bush, and also, I think, often to the fact that many grown men had very young girl brides, many females had been badly injured and had been left with fistulas – that is holes, into either bladder or rectum, sometimes into both, with very unpleasant results which were almost impossible to cope with as may be imagined, yet these poor girls and women had to live with the disgusting sequelae of their injuries. How they coped with it all goodness only knows, and they would come to the clinic in sheer desperation. The only answer was surgery and I would try to get them away to Kano if I could where I knew there was a consultant available. However, not everyone could manage to travel so far – for to do so cost money, and transport was difficult in any case. Who could afford to fly? Few had cars available. Most people travelled on foot or by donkey, and you never saw women riding donkeys – they would be expected to trudge behind their husbands who rode the animal. I only once saw a woman being brought into hospital by her husband who had lifted her onto the donkey while he walked because she was so ill. I have seen women literally crawling across to the clinic because they were too weak to walk. If women could not get to any other hospital far away, then we simply had to do what we could in the way of surgery ourselves. Many a time I have spent my breakfast hour with my surgical textbook open in front of me, revising what I was going to have to do when I went into theatre straight afterwards. What alternative was there?

The ever present numbers of people waiting to be seen meant that the medical and expatriate nursing staff often didn't finish their 'working day' until long after everyone else did. However, that is the nature of our jobs and none of us ever felt that we would do otherwise. The working day ended officially at 2 p.m. for most people. After that the thing to do was to have a quick lunch – and then the bliss of siesta and a bit of a sleep if you were lucky. I usually did a quick ward round before leaving the hospital just to make sure all was quiet. Louis (or I if I was in charge when he went out bush touring) would also pop back to the office to clear the desk for the last time that day before going home.

Until I had my house in order, I did not manage to take a siesta, for I was still busy in my spare time getting on with the interminable curtain making. But as soon as this job was done and the curtains hung, I was more than glad to get on to my bed and sleep for an hour after lunch. In the UK, the idea of an hours' kip every afternoon would be comical, but in the tropics it can be a life-saver, or at the least, an energy saver.

At some stage during the week, one had to fit in a visit to the canteens (shops and supermarkets to you), in order to lay in supplies. One's cook was given 'market money' each week, with which he would buy basics in the African market – meat, any vegetables available (usually not much in the way of fresh vegetables – a few beans, carrots perhaps, okra, potatoes) and he would buy flour and eggs. Houseboys, although supplied by their employers with 'uniform' – working outfits, one for daytime, and a white one for evening, generally wore their own clothes when going to market, for, they said, if the stall holders realised they were buying supplies for expatriates, the price would go up alarmingly. The amount of market money was arbitrary. I would give my cook a set amount each week. He never asked me for more, and I never asked for anything back in the way of change. It worked out, I think, to the satisfaction of us both. At the canteens one did not find fresh foods. Everything was tinned or bottled or powdered and in packets or other containers. I would, for instance, buy Klim, which was a Dutch powdered milk. When made up, it really did taste like real milk and I drank quite a lot of it.

You had to make time to get to the canteens, for they too closed at the normal end of the working day, so I would try to leave work early once a week and dash to what was called 'The Beach' to do my shopping before everything closed. 'The Beach' was an old term, arising, I was told, from the early days of trading, when ships came into ports carrying goods. Traders from up country as well as from coastal areas would congregate on the front to see what goods had been brought, what they could buy to sell on from their own stores, as well as what local produce they could in turn sell for export. They would say, when a ship was due, that they were going to the beach to see what was there. The name stuck, and even in Maiduguri, a thousand miles up country from Lagos and the sea, the term survived and was used by some of the older 'old coasters' when going to the local canteens.

I had been told when I first went out that I could make a huge order for dry goods from a firm in Lagos, and that many people did in fact order what they thought they would need for the whole of their tour. I did make such an order once, and it certainly arrived safely, but when I realised that except for certain delicacies I could get most of what I wanted in Maiduguri, I didn't bother doing so again. Another Lagos facility was the supplying of 'cold stores' – that was frozen goods. Again at first, I ordered things like butter or fish or meat from the cold store suppliers. These things were sent up from Lagos by plane, perhaps once a fortnight. However, as they first had to be off loaded at the airport, and then delivered to the hospital office, they were usually thawing by the time I actually got them, and although we stuck them in the fridge at home immediately, and indeed I enjoyed the occasional meal of 'fresh' plaice, I was never quite happy about their state of hygiene (and didn't much like liquid butter anyway) so I soon stopped ordering and managed with what I could get locally for the rest of my time overseas – if tinned butter and cheese were all I could get, and they were, then so be it . The only problem one might have with the local canteens was if, as occasionally happened, one dashed down for essential supplies, only to find closed doors and a big notice saying 'Sorry, Stocktaking'.

After siesta, I would sit out on my verandah, drinking yet more cups of tea until I felt fully re-hydrated, and then, with luck, my time was my own for a few hours. I would read, or write, or occasionally would visit the club library, and maybe have a quick dip in the club's small swimming pool – we had one for adults and a smaller shallower one for the children. The club was a good meeting place because we all went there. The library was not large, but adequate – until you had read all its books, that is. One of the expats was in charge and she tried to get fresh books when they could be afforded from club funds. If anyone had any spare books, these could be presented to the little

41

library too. One could play snooker or billiards, or even in some stations, tennis. There would be evening social functions sometimes – any excuse for something a bit different was welcome – we used to have, for instance, lovely Halloween parties, New Year parties, and so on. Or you could just go for a half hour to see other faces, chat to friends, have a drink. And on Sunday mornings at Maiduguri Club there was always a queue of expatriate men waiting to have their hair cut, for one of the African barbers from the town had learnt to cut European hair (many of the locals had their heads shaved, or had it cut short and 'partings' shaved into it). Alhaji Barber, as he was known to us all, would set up his chair out in the club compound, and the men would in turn take their place there and be trimmed tidily. It was luxury to have such a barber for there were not any in many stations. After I was married and we were posted elsewhere, I was dismayed to find that I would have to cut my new husband's hair. All I had at the time was a small pair of embroidery scissors, and with these I did my best, while he screamed for an anaesthetic! I never believed that my efforts were as painful as that!

In the evenings I would go down to the hospital again to make what I hoped might be the last visit of the day, and I'd check all the wards again to make sure that all was well and that treatments were being properly given, before returning home and sinking into a bath and then changing into fresh clothes. None of us ever used our hot water geysers, for electricity was extremely expensive. Instead, the steward would heat up a metal bucket full of water on top of the cooking stove, and when you were ready, this would be poured into the bath for you, so that you could top it up from the cold water tap and have a bit of a soak. Often, the water from the tap was pretty warm too, because the tanks were in the roof space, so they warmed up through the day anyway.

Unless any emergencies came in after that, I would be free to socialise, provided, if it was my turn on call, that I could be contacted somehow if a call came. As I have said, few people had telephones, so that I couldn't leave an alternative contact with the nursing staff. This meant that unless my house-boys could run round to where I had gone, I would refuse invitations on my on-call weeks. If I was not out for dinner, then I had a quiet meal at home, and would sit outside afterwards, enjoying the cool of the night, and reading, or writing letters – or even doing nothing more than just sitting and taking in the peace and tranquillity, the dark velvet sky and the stars.

And that was the pattern of my day.

Chapter 6

The hospital, as mentioned earlier, had several wards all built as separate blocks, each fitted out as Nightingale wards. Most beds, therefore, were in the main long room, at one end of which was a tiny office for the nursing staff. Beyond this was a small side ward with two or three beds in it, for very ill patients, or sometimes for any regarded as 'important people' in the local community – local councillors for instance. Most patients would be in proper beds, but others had to sleep on mattresses or sleeping mats if all the beds were full. These would be placed on the floor between beds, or even out on the surrounding verandahs unless it was the rainy season. There were almost always lots of extra people present as well – family and friends, some of whom might bring their own sleeping mats to use at night, though we did try to persuade them to go home at night.

Equipment varied a lot. In the ante room to the operating theatre was a glass fronted cupboard holding spare instruments. I remember thinking when I looked at these that some of them might not have been used for years, if at all. They certainly had not been looked after. One of the first things I had to try to do in theatre was to plate a fractured radius and ulna. Yes, there were the requisite instruments and a few small plates of different sizes in the cupboard – even some screws. But I had to pick and choose very carefully and discard the rusty ones before I could do anything. Very luckily I had been given a few surgical instruments to bring with me from the hospital in Beverley where I had been working previously. These I kept at my house and only brought them to the hospital if I needed to do so. They were very precious items for me and I guarded them like a dragon guards its horde.

I think what I treasured most of all was my supply of syringes – old glass ones which the Beverley hospital no longer used, as plastic disposable ones had recently become the order of the day there. Even more precious was my supply of needles of various sizes to use with the syringes – for nobody looked after such things in Maiduguri – or indeed anywhere else in Nigeria where I had worked, except to wash and sterilise them by boiling. We had no facilities for sharpening needles, and with the rather rough handling that they got, they soon became hooked at the end, or otherwise blunted, and injections were then difficult to give. I looked after my own needles and syringes very carefully and never allowed anyone else to touch them. I had my own portable steriliser too, so on the whole I managed to keep them in fairly good nick throughout each tour of duty, and replaced them each time I went to the UK on leave. They usually just about lasted out for a tour.

The nursing staff varied. The charge nurses and senior theatre staff had all had some training, though none of it as comprehensive as it would have been in the UK. Many, if not most of the others had not been trained at all at that time, though Matron was trying to do some regular teaching to provide something in the way of training, occasionally asking Louis and me to do some teaching when we had time.

Some of the nurses in fact were not literate at all, although they could speak English, but others only spoke their own language – Hausa or Kanuri (sometimes both). I was warned to keep a good eye open to make sure that patients really did get the treatment I had prescribed, for there were some nurses who would demand payment from patients before they would give medicines or bedpans, or even drinks of water. This sort of thing was a way of life there very often, but had to be controlled when it came to health care – if possible.

It was clear to me that I must learn to speak Hausa in order that my patients could talk to me directly, knowing that I could understand them, rather than going through an interpreter, who could of course tell me anything. I hasten to say here that I think most of the senior staff were probably quite honest, but from time to time one did find otherwise, sometimes in the most surprising areas. I have already mentioned how Matron dealt with empty penicillin phials so that they could not be refilled with water that was probably unsterile and then sold on in the town. We always had a number of patients turning up as outpatients with huge abscesses on the outer sides of their thighs, or in the buttocks, that we felt had come from having had dirty injections given to them by native 'doctors' in the town.

On this subject, I was once summoned to the Court House on the GRA to speak to one of the High Court judges who was visiting that week to try various cases which couldn't be dealt with by the local native courts. I waited in an ante room until his current session ended, and he came through to see me, stripping off his hot red robes and heavy wig thankfully before reaching out for a long cool drink. Then, "Will you look at the contents of this bag," he said, "and tell me which preparations would be dangerous if not used properly?" A huge leather bag was put onto the table in front of me. I opened it, to find inside an enormous collection of medicines of all kinds – bottles of variously coloured liquids, packets of all kinds of tablets, and vials of all sorts of preparations for injection, penicillin, stibophen, morphia and so on and so on.

I gave the only possible answer, which was "Any medicine if not properly used can be dangerous. You have to be sure that whoever prescribes it is properly trained, likewise whoever administers these things. If they get into the wrong hands and are illegally and improperly used, they can do great harm."

The haul had been found in a house in Maiduguri where the occupants had no training or authority whatever in medicine or nursing or any other form of health care. All the medicines had been stolen, were probably for onward sale and many would have been adulterated in some way. The case was to come up in court later that week, and I was asked to attend to give my statement, while the bag and its contents would be used as evidence. I had been amazed to see just how much was in that bag – and what a variety of preparations were there. I hoped they had not all come from our hospital pharmacy or wards.

Back to the nursing staff. Our old midwife, Hadja was, so far as I could gather, untrained. But she had been there for so many years and had picked up an enormous amount of wisdom through experience and had learnt from the many doctors with whom she had worked. We all had confidence in her, and knew that matters were safe in her hands. She knew exactly when she needed to call one of us. She never tried to deal with anything 'different' herself, although she usually knew what would be needed, and anticipated well. By the time one of us had arrived if she had called, Hadja would have got everything ready so that no time would be lost. It would be a bad day for the hospital when she eventually retired, and I hoped that this wouldn't be in my time there. The expatriate nursing staff were all trained and experienced midwives, so that they kept a close eye on the maternity unit as well. It was really very well served.

The theatre staff were also very good – the senior ones, that is. They too did not have full training as we know it here in the UK, but they did have some simple instruction in anatomy and nursing care, and the rest, once again, they had learnt from successive medical officers over the years. Mallam Maidugu Biu was the nurse in charge, and he would 'take' the operations, acting as assistant to the doctor, or second assistant if we ever had the luxury of two of us being scrubbed up together. He was excellent, calm and unflappable, clean and particular about the way in which he dealt with everything. The next in seniority, Mallam Ajiya, was also good, though a very different personality from Maidugu Biu. He would give the anaesthetics. In spite of the fact that he would not have had anything like the training in this skill that I had received when a student, he was remarkably able and gave a good 'dope'. When one considers that the anaesthetic of choice there at that time was rag and bottle chloroform, this was an amazing achievement. Chloroform is known to be more risky for the patient than ether (which we also had), nevertheless it was safer than ether to have around the place, because it was not flammable. In the hot climate, ether was not used unless for some reason chloroform could not be used. I might also add that ether seems to cause much more bleeding, and as we had no means of transfusion at all, anything which caused as little bleeding as possible was favoured. The consequence of all this was that not only did the doctor have to cope with the actual surgery, but at the same time he had to keep a close eye on the anaesthetic too, in case anything did seem to be amiss. During my time there I had to deal with some quite difficult cases in theatre, and our nurse-anaesthetist really coped wonderfully well every time. It was the same in another station where I worked too. However, when both Louis and I were in station at the same time, and if the operation in hand was not too complex, then I would handle the rag and bottle and chloroform instead. Kept me in practice if nothing else, though I knew that I would never be required to do it back in the UK – anaesthesia had moved on and was several light years ahead by then.

We had to do a lot of 'make do and mend' in the hospitals I worked at in those days. I was constantly having to scrape the barrel for orthopaedic equipment when I tried to set up various forms of traction for fractures. Louis would pull my leg (no pun intended) over it, and vowed he would set up a special orthopaedic ward for me.

Apropos of orthopaedics, I remember one really funny moment, though I didn't dare laugh when it happened. I was fixing a man with a fractured femur on to traction. I had set up a Balkan Beam, and we were putting his leg first of all into a Thomas' splint. For the uninitiated, this treatment means that initially you have to put various strips of strapping onto and round the leg, so that from its end, once in the splint, a weight can hang which will ensure that the fractured bones are kept in the proper position however much the patient moves about in bed. It is in the end a system of pulleys and cords. To start with, and before we could fix the splint on, somebody had to hold the leg by the ankle and heel, keeping a steady pull on it in order to maintain the set position while somebody else applies the strapping. I would do the strapping myself because it was important to have it just right, so I asked one of the nurses to hold the leg and to keep the steady pull on it for me. This can be a pretty hard task if you simply stand up straight and try to pull hard – and you do have to pull hard. However, I had always been taught that you could save yourself a lot of effort and fatigue if you let yourself lean back so that your own body weight acted as part of the 'pull'. You could then concentrate largely on holding the leg in position, which was vitally important.

I explained this to the nurse, who had clearly been struggling to stand straight, pull with some power and at the same time keep the leg in position.

It seemed so easy to me, having done it myself so many times in previous years. He couldn't get the idea at all, and was rapidly wearing himself out. Again I urged him to do as I suggested and explained all over again carefully what I wanted him to do.

"But doctor!" he expostulated, "I cannot do this. I have had ten children you see!"

Forbearing to ask, "and what about your poor wife in that case?" I had to contain my amusement and just get on with it as best I could.

In an effort not to waste anything, bandages were washed and re-used quite often because we never seemed to have enough stock, and we used a lot of dressings because there were so many tropical ulcers to deal with. These could be huge, crippling and sometimes life threatening. Even in our own houses we recycled just about everything. I never threw away any paper or string – even newspapers were kept, and I would spend a lot of time untying knots in string if I had any parcels sent to me. Everything was precious. Squash bottles, once empty, were cleaned and kept for water storage – we used gallons of water for drinking and one of the cook's main tasks was to keep the supply going. Our house-boys kept all empty food tins, which they could use as oil lamps, putting a little oil into the empty tin and something to act as a wick, or they would be used as candlesticks. There being no street lights, if we were expecting guests in the evenings, we would make a sort of flare path along both sides of the drive with candles stuck in small empty food tins. As we only had rain or wind during one part of the year, candles never went out because of the weather during the other months. They looked very pretty when used in this way.

Although I wasn't really too bothered by the heat and found that I could work quite quickly in it, I realised how hot it was simply from the state of my clothes, which always seemed to be sodden with sweat. How glad I was of my cotton garments. All the information sent to me had indicated that only cotton would be suitable, and how right that was. Dresses, bras, panties, petticoats – I'd bought everything in cotton. Petticoats, in fact, I never wore anyway – they made me far too hot. In time, everything would wear out, rotted by sweat as well as by the action of the sunlight when hung out on the line to dry after being washed. I particularly found that the bits of my bras with the hooks and eyes on them went first and I was for ever writing home to ask my mother if she could get hold of bra repair kits to send out to me – they were impossible to find where I was.

I'd managed to buy about five cotton dresses to take out, but two of those had to be kept to wear if I was going out in the evening. I quickly realised that the remaining three would not keep me going for very long, so I started to patronise a shop in the town run by an Arab trader, who had a great variety of materials from which to choose. Many of the local women bought rather exotic stuffs – gauzy fabrics, even Lamé sometimes. However, there was a reasonable selection of cottons too. I discovered that we could order (through the Club librarian) paper patterns from Lagos, so I chose and ordered a pattern for a plain all-purpose, very easy-to-make dress, and a ditto blouse. As soon as they arrived my work was, literally, cut out and once again, using my trusty little sewing machine, I made several frocks and blouses – all in exactly the same shapeless style, but at least of different colours and prints. With a belt on, the dresses were passable – but I was never a dressmaker, and looked forward to a time when somewhere I could replenish my wardrobe with more exciting garments. My mother, realising the situation, sent lengths of dress material to me as well, from time to time. If not stylish, at least I was able to keep decently clad.

In addition to the hospital, there were outlying bush dispensaries. These were small clinics consisting of mud or breezeblock buildings, sited in remote areas of the provinces. They were staffed by very simply trained dispensary attendants who did what they could in the way of health care for the local populace. Some of them were very good indeed. They were supplied with a certain amount of equipment – bandages and dressings, medication for various common ailments, including treatments which had to be given by injection. In order to be allowed to give injections, the attendants had to have 'injection licences'. A licence meant that you had been taught how to give certain injections, and your licence stipulated exactly what you were allowed to give in this way. If you only had a licence which allowed you to give penicillin, for instance, then you were only allowed to give that and not anything else via a syringe. So you could treat pneumonia, but not bilharzia, for example. Some of the dispensary attendants had licences allowing them to give several kinds of injection treatment, others did not.

The dispensaries had to be examined by one of the doctors every year, and on the results of that inspection (a report always had to be sent in to the Ministry in Kaduna) depended the renewal of the annual grant in aid for that clinic. The dispensary attendants knew that if there was an adverse report, the clinic would be closed and their jobs lost, so they did try to run things properly. As I said, some were very good indeed. They were required to keep good records and to keep the clinics and supplies in good order. All this meant, therefore, that in addition to running the local hospital, we also had to fit in bush touring.

We did this during Harmattan. Harmattan was our 'winter' season, when nights could be quite cold and we would enjoy the luxury of snuggling under a blanket when we went to bed. There was no rain then and the roads were dry and passable. The Harmattan wind blew dust in from the desert – dust that sometimes was so thick in the air that it blotted out the landscape. Mosquitoes disappeared and many people dispensed with mosquito nets for a few weeks.

Chapter 7

My boys and I soon shook down into a good working relationship. I began to feel that I could trust most of the people I worked with at the hospital, and started to realise the worth of the senior clerk in the office – a good clerk (and there were many) was worth his weight in gold. They were almost always Southern Nigerians, or men from the Middle Belt. Mr Sofosu, our clerk, must have been very patient with me at first, I think, giving me time to learn about his country and people, during which I am sure I was very impatient and perhaps rather prickly at times. I think he probably began to approve of me when they found that I was taking Hausa lessons and could start to speak to patients directly in the clinics – for he told me that the office staff thought I had learnt to do so very quickly – and they had obviously given me several Brownie points for my efforts.

Samuel, my cook-steward, and Amadu, my small boy, got together as a team, and (especially after I had once had an unexpected day off, at which time I had gone round the house myself with dustpan and brush, dusters and polishes, showing them exactly how I liked everything to be done) – they kept the whole place spick and span. There was a protocol amongst one's houseboys, and they did not overstep each other's duties while keeping the household ticking over nicely. Only occasionally did I ever hear of disagreements between staff, and was lucky never to have had such situations to cope with myself.

I have described how I would give my cook an allowance of market money each week with which he bought basics from the local market. The small boy also had a tiny allowance (it was about sixpence a week when I was there), and with this he bought charcoal for the iron. One of his jobs was to do the washing and ironing. Few of us had electric irons – if you were posted to a station without electricity, what use would they be anyway? If anyone did have one, she used it herself and didn't let it anywhere near the boys. They all used charcoal irons extremely well. These irons, which I have only ever seen in museums in the UK, where they were considered to be anachronisms, were in general use in 'my' part of Nigeria. The locals called them 'pressing stones', which suggests to me a much earlier method of getting creases out of newly washed clothes.

Samuel soon discovered that I was by inclination a vegetarian (I have no principles about meat, it's just that I never liked it much) – so he made me wonderful omelettes for my evening meals. I think he really wished sometimes that I would start to entertain guests, for he seemed to enjoy cooking, and he must have been very bored with looking after somebody who not only ate very little anyway, but who was also content with a very simple, perhaps monotonous diet.

This was brought home to me one day when I asked him if there was anything he specially wanted me to get from the canteens, and his hopeful reply was "If you can get baking powder, Madam, in case strangers come and I have to bake food quickly."

It was clearly time for me to start to return all the hospitality I had been given!

As yet, I only had the crockery and cutlery I'd brought out to Nigeria – a small set of four placings, so at first I could only invite a very few people at a time, but once I started to be paid, I was able to buy more tableware, and gradually I could have more people in together. It was surprising how quickly the list grew of people I wanted to invite back. Although we worked for long hours, Louis and I, we did have time for a good social life as well – in fact I had more social activities than I'd ever had in my life before.

In England, I had recently learned to ride, and while always being nervous of horses, I adored riding so long as I could be with somebody. I discovered that we were at that time allowed to ride the local police horses at the end of the day – they were 'off duty' then, and probably hadn't had much exercise during the day so were ready to go out. I was invited to join a small group of other expats whenever I wanted, so once or twice a week, with Louis taking calls for me, I met them at about 5 p.m. when we all turned up at the stables and had an hour's riding, that is, until it got dark which was just after 6 p.m. There was really no twilight that far south, either it was daylight, or it was dark all in about fifteen minutes. My horse, like all the others, was quite small as compared with the animals we see here at home:

'The General Hospital
Maiduguri
1.10.1957

...They are all stallions, nobody ever rides mares, & the horses are never gelded, so they are extremely energetic & full of zip. The one I ride is a lovely little chestnut, he gleams gold & almost has a yellow-green sheen in some lights. He has a nice little head & neck & is a lovely mover & very very fast when he is really trying to catch somebody else up, but so far has been very well behaved with me, though he has been known to bolt. He gets a little bit excited if he sees the others start to gallop.

He is called No. 39 – they are all known by their numbers, & none of them are used to sugar & don't know what to do with it!

I've been out on him twice now. We go off through the bush in a big circle. Yesterday we didn't get back till after dark...

...But we seem to gallop nearly all the way – these animals could go for ever & not be tired, I think! The native saddles are very high back & front far more than ours. And they ride with very long stirrups which I find uncomfortable so I take my own stirrup leathers now.

Everybody rides here – the natives, I mean – they ride patient little donkeys, which are also used as pack animals & my goodness they earn their keep too!

They ride horses – and the Kanuri women, that is the local tribe – are allowed to ride by their menfolk, which is rather unusual as in Nigeria the women do the fetching & carrying usually while the men take it easy – but they don't ride horses they ride oxen and bulls! The bulls I must say look very placid but they are only harnessed with bits of twine & they are enormous – I'd never dare to go near one I'm sure!'

When we rode out, we often used a dry riverbed as our bridle path – but that was only possible in the dry season. The surface was very uneven, with often large potholes and pools, so you had to keep a good look out not to be brought down by them. We all enjoyed riding and were very sorry to be told a few months later that the horses would not be available any more as they were going on patrol out of station. Later on I had the use of an ex-race horse, by name Market Boy. He was wonderful to ride, and I would go out on him alone sometimes, as well as together with others. But sadly in the end he was a bit too strong and frisky for me – no wickedness, just high spirits, but I had to give him up. A pity.

Work-wise I settled in to my routine, and domestically I soon felt as though I had lived this way all my life. The house ran smoothly. We were very privileged on the GRA to have running water and electricity – almost all the time, anyway. Electricity was very expensive, so that although we were all happy to use it for lighting and for our ceiling and table fans, almost nobody had electric fridges, and nobody ever used the hot water geysers in the bathrooms.

The only people who had – and used – air conditioners were the commercial folk, for such things were provided and paid for by the firms for which they worked. And nobody ever used, or even had provided, electric cookers when I first went out. Fridges were run on kerosene, and mine seemed to be perfectly efficient, though I know I was lucky, as some regularly broke down.

Cooking was done on a wood stove, for which you bought a cord of wood, which had to be chopped up – but you would hire labour for just a day, perhaps two days, for the chopping to be done. A cord of wood cost thirty shillings, and looked to be an enormous amount. Once chopped up, it was stacked up in a lockable wood store room if you had one, or in your garage if not, so that none would be stolen. It was not until several years later that we graduated to a gas cooker for which I would have to go to the canteens for cylinders of calor gas. Most of the cooks preferred to use the wood stoves, actually, and they could manage in all sorts of other ways if they had to. My cook Ali (who came to me after Samuel left, and who stayed with me until I retired permanently from Nigeria) could bake bread in a cut-down kerosene tin if necessary when we were out on tour and in a bush rest house.

Each evening your boys would heat a zinc bucket of water on the stove, which would then be poured into the bath for you. Actually in some places, water would be almost too hot to use when it came out of the tap. The house water supply came straight from the roof tank. Theoretically it was cold water, but because during the day the corrugated pan roofs would heat up, the tank also heated, so you never expected to get cold water from the taps, and indeed you didn't. If a house had an electric geyser, you could use the 'hot' tap, but one could not cool the hot water down because the 'cold' taps only produced warm water anyway. In any case, as indicated, we didn't use our geysers as electricity was so costly. At all other times of the day, cold water rather than hot was what we wanted, and in fact, once I had washed in the morning when I got up, I refilled the bath so that it would have had time to cool for when I got back home at the end of the working day – if, that is, the boys had not needed to use it all earlier. Why should they? Well, because the water was more often than not cut off during the day, so we found that shortly after I had got away to work, there would be nothing coming from the taps until evening. So we all had to rely on what was stored in the bath. The boys would probably have managed to get the day's laundry done in it just before the water supply was cut off. Laundry was always done in the bath – we didn't have washing machines. The rule was that whenever the water in the bath had been used, everyone made sure to either refill or top up if the supply had not already been cut off, so that we always had some available.

Electricity would also very often be cut off, and this could happen at night too, so one always kept a supply of candles and matches at the ready. At the hospital, we could be taken by surprise if we were working in theatre when supplies were cut off, as we had no emergency lighting or water supply. So in Maiduguri we always started very early in the day if we could. Otherwise one might not be able to scrub up, nor use the theatre light. In remote outstations, where there was no electricity anyway, surgery had to be done by the light of Tilley lamps. Thankfully I was never in that position, for it would have made theatre unbearably hot to work in.

One of the things I enjoyed very specially was sitting out on my verandah after I'd had my evening meal and finished my hospital night rounds. It was dark, cool, and very quiet. There was a pretty creeper growing round the verandah, called coralita, which had a tiny pink flower. The light shining on it from my lounge turned the leaves a pale delicate creamy green, and it looked lovely against the velvety sky. How peaceful it was to sit there, and if I was not going out, I would spend a lot of time there, just sitting and looking – and surprisingly for me, not even feeling the need to read. The only sounds to be heard would be those of the cicadas and mosquitoes – and also what I felt was part of life in Africa – the fact that there always seemed to be the sound of padding feet. No matter what time of night you happened to be up, somebody was always going somewhere. Barefoot walking on sand has a sound all of its own. If I was called out in the small hours, I was always sure that the footsteps were those of the 'thief-men' I had so often been warned about. More likely, in fact, they would be house-boys who had been out for the evening after their work for the day was done. There was a magic about those soft warm black nights – different from anything else I had known.

In my compound were some big neem trees, one of which was just outside the verandah. When, during my first evenings there, I saw big flying things coming and going, and heard all sorts of chirruping and squawky sounds, a bit like Donald Duck, I thought they were birds. Gradually I realised that they were fruit bats coming and going from their roost in the tree. They would swoop in noisily, and then fold themselves up very small and there was silence as they hung from their branches and slept. Lots of people, I discovered, had bats in their roof spaces, with bat droppings eventually giving the show away. Possibly my house was the same. The bats, and the ever present lizards which came and went at will into and around the house accounted for many of the nocturnal 'house noises' that I heard after I went to bed. Yes, the silence at night was really quite a loud silence, but one which made you feel totally alone in a huge world – and very content.

Once I'd had my evening meal, I would let my boys go off duty – it was nice to feel that I had the house to myself. I locked the back door after they had gone, but only locked the front door when I went to bed – until then one left doors and windows open for coolness. And here is something quite typical of Africa – Nigeria anyway.

Dr Simpson had pointed out to me that my front door lock did not function. A large hasp and staple had been put on to it so that they could be padlocked and the house secured – but they had been fixed on the outside of the door.

In order to lock the front door, therefore, I had to go outside, and then get back into the house by the back door. Here was another problem, for the back door lock was also faulty. It only worked from the inside. When, therefore, I wanted to lock up for the night, I had to unlock the back door and go outside to the front, there locking the padlock, and returning to the back door to get inside again, before locking that on the inside. If I was called out in the night, I had to unlock the back door, run round to the front, unlock the padlock, go inside and through to the back door which I then locked from inside, before finally going out through the front door, locking the padlock again once I was outside, and then getting into my car to drive down to the hospital. The whole process had to be done in reverse on my return home before the house was finally re-locked and secure again. And of course, I always had to be up in the morning before my boys arrived, so that I could open the back door (from the inside) to let them in. Dr Simpson told me that he had reported this to the Public Works Yard on many occasions but that nothing had every been done about it.

Some months later I had the Yard Superintendent, Bill Martin, and his wife, Mary, in for dinner. Bill noticed the padlock and asked why I had put it on – thinking no doubt that I was a scared cat and no mistake. He had it all sorted out in a very short time and how nice it was to be able to open, shut and lock my doors like other people. Saved a lot of hassle. It could only happen in Africa!

At this point, a few quotations from my original letters might prove useful. It may be that, being written at the time, they come over as very fresh and therefore transmit better my impressions and reactions as I gradually adjusted to the colours, people, culture and so on.

Extracts from letters written between 8.10.57 and 14.10.57:

'Temperature – today, this afternoon, in my bedroom, 90° in the shaded room – that is with curtains drawn. It's much hotter outside of course. In spite of it, I sleep soundly in siesta...'

'...a visit from my next door neighbour who has just returned from a weekend at Fort Lamy, over in French territory, & who has brought me some apples! The first apples I've seen since coming here, & a real luxury.
The fruits at the moment here are fresh grapefruit, oranges & bananas. The grapefruit are lovely very juicy & sweet – & green, with almost pink flesh, not at all like the ones we have at home.
Soon we will be able to get vegetables for a month or two, & then there

won't be any more for several months & we shall have to live on tinned ones if they are obtainable, & vitamin tablets.'
[I never did take vitamin tablets – we all seemed to stay healthy without]

'Next question – what I wear – answer – as little as possible! I couldn't bear a petticoat.'
[I would wear bra and pants and a cotton dress, or skirt and blouse – we didn't have T-shirts in those days]

'I'll not reply [to your letter] in detail, for one thing I've only just got home (3 pm) – which is about 3 hours later than one hopes for, & I seem to have been in & out of theatre all day & am boiling hot & wringing wet! I've done my first big amputation...'

'We also have a couple of hyenas on the station – I think I saw one in my compound the other night & was petrified – but my doors were shut & anyway everyone assures me that they are very cowardly animals & all you do is make a sudden loud noise (a scream?) & off they go. I hope so!'

'It has been very hot again today – we had a cool day last week which was very nice – I even wore my slacks & a cardigan one afternoon when I was pottering about – & then when I looked at my thermometer I laughed to see how much the temperature had dropped – from 88° down to 80° [Fahrenheit]. Fancy feeling cool at 80°!'

'I'm getting quite accustomed to surgery now – Louis laughs at me when I say I don't like it, & says, "Well you're not doing so badly for somebody who says they can't operate!" So I suppose he isn't too horror stricken by my efforts.'

'I can't think what I want for Christmas – the only thing I'm really lacking in the house is a lavatory brush, but it is such a queer thing to ask for!'

'The insects do make an enormous noise here – I can hear bangings & crashings outside on the verandah, due to a large dragonfly bashing its way around, & there is a cricket which sits in the kitchen sink at night & sings very loudly. And there is a cockroach in the bathroom & another in the lavatory which come out at nights only. They are quite companionable, and if they aren't there at night, I almost wonder what's happened to them!

There are also little toads which live outside & they quite often hop into the lounge at night if you are sitting with the door open.

The lizards intrigue me – they are lovely little things, all different colours...& they play all day long – some are green with orange heads, some are black & green & yellow stripes, some are just a porridge-colour – that sort usually live in the house on the walls, & are good because they eat insects, but the boys think they are very poisonous & are terrified of them. I came in one day to find the curtains down & Samuel & Amadu chasing one of these poor little things with a big stick in a panic. Samuel said, "It's poisonous, like snake." So I said, "Well, let it live in peace". So rather sheepishly they went back to the kitchen, & I heard Samuel say to Amadu "Well, anyway, there is a doctor here!" '

Chapter 8

Which Doctor?

No, I haven't spelt the above incorrectly. It is just that I sometimes wondered quite what my role was.

I didn't meet any witch doctors face to face – perhaps there were not so many in Northern Nigeria as in the Southern and Eastern Regions. There were, however, a number of 'native doctors' (so described to me by the locals), who were also spoken of as either Kanuri doctors or Hausa doctors. Some of them clearly had good basic ideas, but when translating them into action, might produce very varying results, some of them disastrous. I had, in the years before going overseas, read stories of strange happenings in far-off places in magazines like 'The Wide World'. Once I knew that I was going to West Africa, I recalled vivid descriptions of 'Leopard men' for instance. These stories, I was later to learn, were based on experiences in Nigeria, but mostly in the Southern parts of the country.

On our long drive from Maiduguri to Lagos years later when we were going on our retirement from the country, I felt that I knew why such practices were rife in those more southerly areas, for as one left the open savannah and orchard bush of the North and came into the lush forested parts, I felt a very oppressive sense of almost menace as the road twisted in and out of the dense growth. In the North you could generally see the road ahead for some distance. But here, in the rain forest, and because the road had to curl and twist round so much, you could often not see further than the next bend, giving a feeling of being trapped by the terrain and vulnerable to watching eyes. You would drive for many miles, sometimes in quite dark shade from the huge trees, yet there was often the feeling that somebody had just slipped quickly out of sight into the undergrowth. This gave me the idea that we were in a country where such claustrophobic vulnerability could very easily be exploited and used to intimidate and terrify people who were only too willing to believe in powerful medicine, or spells, or threats. This would apply to all sorts of situations, not just medical ones.

When I was a small child, a bigger bullying child could threaten you with a horrific image that stayed in your mind, getting ever more awful as time passed. You believed what you were told and the other child therefore gained power over you. It's all the same sort of thing.

I hadn't actually given any thought to this as being something I might come across, and was therefore taken considerably aback when, after only having been in Nigeria for a couple of months at most, I popped into the office one day to see Louis. Seated at his desk, he was regarding with some concern a young woman who was lying on the concrete floor just inside the office door. She was surrounded by about a dozen people who, I gathered, were friends and family members. They had brought her to the hospital, it was explained to me by the senior clerk who interpreted for them, because a spell had been cast upon her. Since then she had not been able to move, nor could she eat, speak or respond in any way to any stimulus. They could see, he went on, that if this state of affairs continued, she would die, which was exactly what the spell caster had said would happen. Therefore they had brought her to the hospital as a last resort for the English doctors to cure. I got this story after Louis had gone, because as soon as I arrived, and with a naughty twinkle in his eye, he had said to me "Oh Kath, I was just going to send a message for you. Could you deal with this? I have to go to the wards." And with that he smartly disappeared. Wondering if she perhaps had some sort of gynaecological complaint, I had asked our clerk, Mr Sofosu, to translate for me while I asked questions and waited for answers – none came.

A dozen pairs of eyes turned to me – in silence.

Everyone waited.

I was totally nonplussed – this was the last thing I had expected. How did one remove a spell?

The girl lay motionless, her face expressionless, her eyes open but not focussing on anything. Had she had an epileptic fit, I wondered. No, it had gone on too long for her to be in a post epileptic trance-like state. Had she had some sort of intracranial catastrophe? She looked well nourished and did not seem to be anaemic.

I got down on my knees on the concrete floor and proceeded to do a full physical examination, head to toe, back to front, side to side, all systems. Everything seemed to be normal – central nervous system, circulatory system, chest, abdomen, skeletal – there was nothing to find which might point to a diagnosis, nothing which suggested any malfunctioning anywhere. Yet she was totally inert and showed no response at all to commands or any other stimulus. Hysteria? Hypnosis? Twelve pairs of eyes still looked at me expectantly – still in silence.

Mr Sofosu hovered in the doorway, also waiting to see what I would do. I knew that I had to do something – and quickly. I took a gamble and trusted to luck that in spite of appearances, this girl could both see and hear and also comprehend. I gambled too on the hope that none of them seemed to have any English, and that Mr Sofosu, our clerk, knew no Shakespeare. Then, removing my stethoscope from round my neck, I ceremoniously straightened it out, and then, with as much solemnity as I could muster, traced patterns with it over the girl's body, while at the same time, declaring, with as much passion as I could summon, Portia's speech in the courthouse from 'The Merchant of Venice', it being the only thing I could call to mind at that moment.

"The quality of mercy is not strained..."

I went through as much of the speech as I could remember, before hanging my stethoscope round my neck again, and said, "The spell is gone. I have sent it away with a more powerful one. Tell her this, and also tell her that she will never be so troubled again. She can get up and go home now. She is cured."

I crossed my fingers while everything was translated for her. I was ready to run for my life if nothing happened, thinking that if she continued to lie there the family would probably lynch me. I hardly dared to hope – until – to my immense relief, she got up, and spoke to her relatives – and they all walked out of the office and went home. The honour of the English doctors had been upheld – and I hoped I had gained a few Brownie points for myself as well.

Another time I was asked to see a woman student who, I was told, had been bewitched by 'iska' – spirits. Iska was also the name for the wind that blows through the trees. This girl was on her bed in the dormitory, moaning and talking a lot of nonsense, and altogether behaving in a very odd way indeed. She was very obviously hysterical, and needed nothing more than a firm talking to, which very soon did the trick.

However, I was to find that 'iska' covered a multitude of syndromes, from being under the influence of a spell to being under the influence of – sometimes – alcohol. Usually such patients were pagans, for Moslems were forbidden to drink alcohol. Sometimes patients were under the influence of toxic substances of the 'magic mushroom' variety. All of these were lumped together as being due to 'iska' – the spirits. Usually a mild sedative was all that was needed for the girls. They were more likely to be hysterical than drugged, because the women's and girls' institutions were always carefully guarded and they were well chaperoned if they went out at all, thus having no chance of misbehaving.

Other things I had to learn about, but in the fullness of time, because they didn't crop up at the start of my time in Nigeria, were nothing to do with magic. They were often genuine treatments given by native 'doctors'. Sometimes local medicine was helpful, sometimes it was not. Often it might be based on sensible ideas which, because of lack of knowledge, were not acted upon in a correct manner. Sometimes the gullibility of people was played on and treatment was more a question of suggestion (like my Portia speech). People were still willing to pay for the 'treatment'. For instance, several years later on, when conducting a school clinic, a boy came to me and said, 'My head has fallen in.' I stared at him. He looked normal enough to me. The dispensary attendant explained:

"He means that he has a headache."

"Then give him some aspirin," was my reply.

"No, that won't do," said the attendant. "It is a Kanuri headache, and can only be treated by a Kanuri doctor in the town. It will cost three pence."

It transpired that if you had a 'Kanuri headache', the only treatment was to see a local medicine man – a native 'doctor' who would push his fingers to the back of your mouth, and then give a great shove upwards on the soft palate. This, it seemed, was where the head had fallen in, and to cure the pain it had to be restored to its proper position. Once that was done, all was well again. The education institutions, the Government schools and colleges had found over the years that it was quicker and more economical to pander to this whole idea, give the student three pence and send him or her off into the town for treatment, rather than to mess about with aspirins and a student who kept to his or her bed for hours, or even days. A nice little earner for the Kanuri 'doctors'. I never managed to beat that treatment with any of my own!

Another symptom that I had to contend with was 'Badema'. This, it seemed, was the beating of the heart. If somebody, usually a boy or a man for obvious reasons, could actually see or feel the impulse of his own cardiac action on his chest wall, he was terrified and thought that he was extremely ill – and would probably die very soon. It seemed to me that a little time and trouble taken to explain what 'Badema' actually was would be well worth the effort. First of all, I would examine people carefully, both palpating the apex beat of the heart (this is what the patient could see and probably feel), as well as listening in with my stethoscope. I would tell the complainants that our hearts beat because we were alive and healthy.

"It's when your heart no longer beats at all," I would say, "that you need to worry. Our hearts are inside our chests [they all knew that of course] – and my stethoscope is what I use to listen to hearts with. If the heartbeat is there, then it means you are alive. If it is there to the front of the chest where you say you can see it, then it is in its proper place and not only are you alive but you are probably healthy as well. Be thankful." I would further explain, "I have also come to know that in slender people, and even in plumper people, it is possible to feel the heartbeat with my fingers, and also in slender people one can see it. That is very reassuring, and from now on, if you can see your

Badema, you should be very pleased, because it means that your heart is beating properly and you are safely alive." I don't know if it helped, but it seemed to do so at the time. We didn't have as many children toddling off to the town for whatever treatment the native 'doctors' thought they could charge to cure *Badema*.

A final example of 'magic' medicine that confounded me was as follows. One of my husband's students came to me one day with some complaint for which he needed an injection. As usual I had brought my own syringes and needles to the clinic, so that I knew they were in good order. I drew up the shot and started to inject. The needle would not, it seemed, penetrate the skin, and I withdrew it to find it was badly hooked. I tried another one – same result.

"It is the medicine," volunteered the student.

"It can't be that," I said "the medicine is perfectly all right for injection."

"No," he replied "I mean it is the medicine I have been given in the town from a Kanuri doctor."

"And what is that?" I asked.

"It is to stop me from being injured by a spear or a knife," he said.

It seemed that he had wanted his skin to be toughened up so that sharp things would not harm him. There were a lot of stabbings in and around Maiduguri, and people seemed to throw spears and such at each other sometimes with gay abandon. Well, whatever had been given to him in the way of 'medicine', it had certainly done the trick. I ruined several hypodermic needles before I was able give him the treatment he needed from me.

Occasionally 'iska' meant an evil influence put upon one by another person. Once when I went on to the children's ward, I found a mother in the process of packing up her child to take it home (mothers usually stayed with their children all the time). The child was really quite ill and nowhere near ready for discharge. I asked the mother what had made her decide to do this. She hesitated at first and then told me angrily and with a little fear too, that the mother of another child in the ward had cast a spell on her. It had not yet taken effect, so she was removing both herself and her child from this evil influence before any serious harm could be done. The other mother, naturally, indignantly refuted this accusation. So in this case, 'iska' was the fact that the other mother was supposed to have summoned up evil spirits (the *iska*) to help her to cast a spell on somebody else. Once again I had to summon up my own brand of 'power' in order to de-activate any bad spell that was floating around, saying firmly that such enchantments knew very well that they had no place in my hospital. Once they were rumbled, I said, they had to depart immediately because they realised that their influence had been destroyed. After that there were no further problems and both mothers stayed put with their respective children.

I am sure there would be many other instances of 'witch doctoring' in Northern Nigeria, but luckily I didn't come across any more myself. What I did notice was that many people carried charms, amulets, whatever one prefers to call them – these took the form usually of a 'charm' written on a piece of paper and tucked into a small leather bag which was worn on a thin leather thong round the neck or on the upper arm. Sometimes I think the 'charms' were short passages from the Koran. All were supposed to protect the wearers from illness or other mishaps.

'Magic' medicine was just another area which nobody at medical school ever told us about. Ah well, I thought, I must just 'brush up my Shakespeare'! I wonder if the old Bard would have smiled if he could have known that not only did he leave the gift of great pleasure to so many people in the theatres of England, but that his words also had a power he would never have imagined over a bewitched young woman in Sub-Saharan Africa some hundreds of years after they were written.

Chapter 9

Although we were always busy, and the outpatient clinics were extremely full and thronged with patients, we knew that equally there were many who did not come for help when they should. The reasons for this were varied. One obvious reason was that of distance. Anyone who lived in the town could easily pop along to the clinics and so long as they were prepared to wait their turn, everyone would be seen that day.

Somebody who was not too ill and who lived in a village anything up to, say, twenty miles away, could and would walk to the hospital. After that, things got difficult. There was no public transport, as we knew it in Britain, at that time. There was a railway system in Nigeria, but not as far as Maiduguri, until a railway was built from Jos to Maiduguri during my last couple of years there – and even then it had not begun to be used. I saw the line completed, and the first railway engine chugging almost as far as Maiduguri itself. From Lagos you could only travel by train as far as Jos. From Kano the only way of getting to us other than by your own efforts was to come by air – and that was financially far beyond the reach of outlying villagers who lived by subsistence farming and only just managed, most of them, to rub along.

There were some kinds of lorry transport – 'Mammy wagons' as they were known. These were almost always overcrowded and often had accidents. One was always being called to the hospital to deal with the results of a Mammy wagon accident, when you could find anything from one or two to a dozen or more injured people lying on the floor of the outpatient clinic, or the ward, or even, as sometimes happened, on the floor of the entrance hall to the theatre, where many would end up during the next few hours. I wrote in one of my letters home regarding Mammy wagons:

'11.11.1957

They are supposed to pass a test of roadworthiness – but it is all a fiddle – for instance they borrow some good tyres, & then as soon as the certificate is given, off come the good tyres & the bad old ones go on again – so of course the trucks come off the roads. And they are always packed to overflowing with Africans, hanging out of the windows & on the running boards.'

A really sick person could not walk easily, if at all. In such cases, people would come on horseback, or donkey back, or in the case of some of the women, on the back of one of the great placid bulls. Occasionally somebody would be brought in by bull-cart, or on a bicycle. One often found that a wife who was ill would be brought by her husband, but that he rode the bike or the donkey, while she had to walk behind. Women in many cases were very much second-class citizens then. I only once actually saw a man bring his wife in and who had lifted her onto his donkey. She was suffering a bad miscarriage and was really far too ill to try to walk. I was thankful, as I expect she was, that he had had the good sense to get her to us as quickly as possible. He got her to us in time, and a few days later she was well enough to be discharged.

Some people really had to travel very long distances to the hospital – occasionally a hundred miles or more. I remember one horrific time when a woman was brought in who had travelled for a couple of days on a cart. She had been pregnant, had gone into labour (in her own village), and then suddenly the baby had impacted when half born and had stuck there. Nobody knew how to help her, and somehow her family got her onto the cart and brought her over tens of miles to us. One can only imagine the agony that poor soul must have suffered on the way, and I was amazed that she had survived the journey. She was in a pretty bad way when she arrived. One's textbooks did not prepare one for this kind of situation, except to mention in the last couple of lines of a chapter that such things used to happen in olden times, but that you should know about them for interest, although they were never likely to happen now. These were the things that came to us all the time. My textbook authors cannot have ever travelled outside the United Kingdom, I sometimes thought! No textbook of mine, even if it mentioned these things as remote complications, ever suggested methods we could employ to deal with them. But deal with them was what we had to do, for there was no other help available. The nearest consultants were at least 400 miles away, and in theory could be contacted by phone. But that contact was not always possible because telephone wires on long empty roads were at times cut and stolen. Wire was useful. Life was not always easy for a general duties medical officer in Maiduguri. Caesarean Section not being possible in this case, I managed with difficulty to complete the delivery of the half-born baby. Sadly, the child was dead, probably having died in its struggle to be born sometime before the mother had left home to come to us. But at least the mother survived, though it was touch and go for a few days. Eventually she was able to return to her village, albeit exhausted after her ordeal. We had all been through a rather anxious time – she, her family and me too, until we knew she was OK again.

Because people had to travel such long distances, and because, therefore, they would delay having to do so until the last minute, trying everything they could think of at home first, it meant that patients often didn't reach us until it was too late, and they died in hospital. This made some people feel that hospital was not a place where you could be cured, but rather it was a place where, if you got there, you would not survive. So they preferred not to come. It was going to take a long time, I thought, for some who lived in remote areas to trust us enough to make the effort to reach us early.

I think that by the time I left Nigeria, more people were realising that they could be successfully treated if they could get to the hospital in good time however, and it was gratifying to think that what you yourself had done was perhaps helping to make a difference to attitudes. The outpatient clinics were always overstretched nevertheless, and I did wonder at times how we could ever have coped with yet more work without having more doctors and fully trained nurses.

Another problem for people travelling from far away was the fact that they had to come to a place where there might be different tribal customs. An extreme case of this was when I once wanted to send a local child to Lagos for specialist treatment. His mother said that she would have to travel with him and stay with him. They could not afford an airfare, so we had to organise Government help for this. Then both mother and child had to undergo some sort of de-tribalisation rite, to enable them to go to the Southern Region, so that took time and complicated things to some extent. Finally we were able to get them on to the plane and away. Neither had been on a plane – in fact I don't think either had even seen one before, so that was a frightening experience for them at first.

Customs and life styles could pose problems. I once had to see a Tuareg woman with a severe gynaecological problem – probably from too much child bearing combined with carrying heavy loads on her head. She and her group had come in from the desert, where they lived a nomadic life, always on the move. I explained to her that an operation was the only way of treating her, and told her that she would have to be careful for some time afterwards, in order for things to heal up and strengthen again. She and her family said they were agreeable. She duly came in and I took her into theatre for the necessary repair. All went well in theatre and she returned to the ward. The next day the family arrived, clearly expecting her to go home with them there and then – she had had her surgery, and so they considered she would now have recovered. Aghast at such an idea, I tried to explain that although the operation had been done, she needed time to heal up and grow strong again, and that she must stay in hospital for a little time longer yet. They understood that wound healing took more than just a few hours, and seemed satisfied.

She progressed, no post-operative complications occurred and she became ambulant a few days later. This, in those days, was really rather quick – I would have preferred her to take things more slowly, and wondered how the internal sutures would stand up to this rate of progress. Then, a day or so later on, the family came back to me again. And this time she was clearly about to leave the hospital with them. I remonstrated, saying that before she could contemplate carrying head loads and doing a lot of walking (their life style meant all of this), she still needed more time for recovery. How about a bit longer? Well, not really, they said – or at least if she herself wished to stay that was up to her – but they would all have moved on by that time, and who knew when they might be back to collect her? They might not be back for as long as two years. She went with them, and the most I could get them to agree to was that they would try not to make her carry head loads for a short time. I have often wondered what became of her.

There was still so much for me to learn. An instance of sheer naiveté on my part when I first arrived was when I suggested to another desert dweller that part of his skin trouble was possibly the fact that he didn't wash thoroughly enough. He looked at me as if I was mad. And then I realised that I was indeed mad to think that a nomadic Tuareg, travelling round the desert could or would waste precious water in frequent washing. The few drops he used for pre-prayer ablutions would be the most he could spare. The rest would have to be used for drinking and, by that means, staying alive. I never made that mistake again.

Although people from outlying areas were reluctant to travel to the hospital, they were very ready to seek our help if we were out on tour. I have explained that outlying dispensaries were our responsibility, and had to be inspected regularly and reported on before their next year's grant in aid was allocated. This meant that as soon as the dry season arrived, one of us went out 'on tour', visiting these districts.

The attendants in the bush dispensaries, as soon as they knew when to expect the doctor, would put the word out, so that when we arrived, there was always a clinic's worth of patients for us to see while we were there. Furthermore, everyone knew where we would base ourselves, and therefore which roads or tracks we would be taking when travelling out each day from base to the various clinics. To save themselves travelling time, many people in these distant areas would make their way from their villages to the road they knew we would take, and we would find ourselves flagged down en route by groups of people waiting to be seen by the doctor. Some of them would have walked, others would have been carried somehow, or would have managed to ride on donkeys. I would be driving happily along a bush track, wondering how many more miles I would have to go before reaching the village to which I was going, when someone would run out onto the track in front of me, waving me down, and then I would see others waiting on the roadside, sitting or even lying on the sand, sometimes in a scrap of shade if there were any nearby trees. How did they know which car to stop? Easy – most of the areas where there were dispensaries were pretty remote, and probably no vehicles would have been seen there for months. When they knew that one of the doctors was due out on tour, then the only car they would see would be the one to flag down.

I would stop the car, get out and spend half an hour trying to take a history and examining the patients as well as I could. Luckily, although by that time I could take a pretty sketchy history in Hausa, I always had either the local Native Authority Health Representative or my cook with me to act as interpreter. Having made a diagnosis, I then had to decide where treatment could best be given. Occasionally I had to say that means should be found to get the person to Maiduguri to the hospital, but more often I knew that the dispensary to which I was going would have the necessary medicines. The dispensaries, although widely scattered, were nevertheless closer to the villages than the hospital in Maiduguri and were therefore much easier for the villagers to reach. If I had known I was going to be consulted on the road, I would have carried a small supply of medicines and equipment with me that first time. Perhaps it was better not to do so in fact, for some 'patients' might well have obtained medicines under false pretences and then sold them on at a huge price. Better that the dispensary attendant saw them and made sure they took their treatment there and then. It was always possible that dispensary attendants, too, might be selling stuff on, but at least there was some control over them because they were required to account in written reports for everything they did and what they handed out as medicine.

The first few months of my overseas service provided an almost perpendicular learning curve professionally for me. I wished that I had been sent on some sort of crash course on medicine in the tropics before going out. Other than having a very sketchy idea of tropical medicine during my student training – and that was mainly simply to tell us to be on the qui vive for malaria in servicemen returning from overseas duty during World War 2 – I had received no teaching of the sort I now wished for.

One thing that did surprise me actually was that I was seeing many ailments in Nigeria that I had seen in Britain as well as tropical ailments. Somehow I had not expected that. It was a surprise when I saw children suffering from things like measles and mumps, and when I found I was treating patients with pneumonia or simple headaches.

Some fifty or sixty miles further up the road from Maiduguri, at a place called Bama, there was a 'Health' doctor. He looked after general public health measures as far as was possible – like organising the supply of smallpox vaccine and arranging for teams of vaccinators to be in place at intervals along the roads, so that they could stop all traffic and vaccinate drivers and passengers in the event of an epidemic starting off. He would send supplies of sulphonamides out to all the villages in the province, to be given out as prophylactics in order to try to prevent the regular outbreaks of meningitis which annually bedevilled the country. And I am sure he would find himself dealing with ordinary clinical problems as well. However, eventually he went on leave, and there was no replacement, at least while I was still doing my initial tour of duty, so that Louis and I took on his duties as well as we could. I remember Louis saying what a headache it was to try to sort out the sulphonamide supply just before the meningitis season, because Bornu was such a huge province and the supply he had received was rather limited.

One huge task which had previously been undertaken by the Health doctor was that of supervising the vaccination against smallpox of pilgrims who were going to Mecca for the annual Hadj. Maiduguri was the main exit point for Mecca in our part of the country, and there were special planes laid on for the pilgrims.

On the outskirts of the town was a pilgrim centre, to which they all had to report. Nobody was allowed to leave the country until they could produce a certificate to say they had been vaccinated against smallpox. Vaccinators were in attendance at the centre, and they were supposed to do the deed and fill in the certificates appropriately. These certificates all had to be individually signed by the medical officer, and the procedure was that a vast bundle of them would be sent to our office, and we would spend an hour signing them all. However, it was not very long before we learned that the vaccinators were accepting 'unofficial' payments for signing certificates without vaccinating (Unofficial payments, did I say? Sweeteners they were), and we were being bamboozled into accepting these as true certification. We changed the whole arrangement forthwith, and, although it meant a much longer time being spent on the task, we said that every pilgrim must attend the hospital in person, passport in hand and arm bared. In that way we could both confirm identity and see the vaccine jelly which had been put on a short time before. Only then would we personally sign the accompanying certificate. At the end of each morning's work, therefore, we took it in turns to go back to the office where there would be a long, long line of people waiting to be inspected. However, chore though it was, we felt that at least we knew things were as all right as we could make them.

The airport authorities had a lot of extra work to do as well, for much supervision was needed in the interests of safety on the planes. When most ordinary people travelled on any form of transport, they would take all their food with them for the journey. I had seen this on the boat with the deck passengers, many of whom had taken stoves with them on which to cook. Again when on the train up country I noticed the same thing. Now, at the airport, many people were embarking once again with food. Some also had small stoves – primus stoves and so on, but sometimes, even worse, some were found trying to light small fires in the aircraft cabin on which to cook en route! To avoid this danger, everyone had to be checked and spoken to before getting on to the aeroplanes. Other problems were those of travel sickness and the results of bodily functions. After the pilgrims had returned to Maiduguri, the word was that the planes were in such a mess that there was no other way to clean them but to remove the seats and hose the whole cabin out completely. All this didn't apply to every traveller – there were those who knew perfectly well how to travel by air.

The chain of command in the Government Health Service was roughly something like this – the general duties medical officers like me were responsible firstly to the doctor who was primarily in charge on the station (for example, in Maiduguri, Louis was in charge and I was his number 2). They would jointly be accountable to the Senior Medical Officer for the province. In our case the senior MO was Bill Moore, who visited us from time to time in the course of his regular tours throughout the province. If he or his family ever reads this I should like to pay tribute here to his good counsel and calm personality. He was a quiet, wise, totally unflappable man of great charm. His wife, Bunny, always travelled with him, and she too was a lovely visitor to have. Nothing seemed to faze them, and however tired or dusty they might be after long exhausting journeys on bad roads, they never let this get in the way of anything. Louis, being my senior, generally entertained them, but just occasionally, if he was out of station, I was more than happy to be able to do so. Above the Provincial Medical Officers were even more senior MO's who would be administrative and based at Governmental level. Above them would be the Minister of Health.

The Minister of Health was, of course a Northern Nigerian. I only met him once. On that occasion he was doing a tour of the Northern Region, visiting hospitals and other administrative health centres. I had been up most of the night trying to cope with an emergency. A man had been shot with an arrow, and had been brought in by lorry from Potiskum, about 160 miles away. The weapon had gone into his eye socket – and he arrived, rather like King Harold, 'with his eye full of arrow'. I feared that the eyeball might have been penetrated. I took him into theatre, and our intrepid nurse anaesthetist did his best with the chloroform while only being able to cover half the face with the mask. Somehow between us we managed to put the man under, and I tried hard to extricate the arrow. Alas it was barbed, and no amount of manipulation on my part would make it shift. Not having anything like a hacksaw available, I couldn't even cut off some of the shaft in order to make things more comfortable for my patient. Despairingly, I had had to send him back to the ward on morphia and antibiotics, and decided to send him on to Kano the next day, to the orthopaedic unit there where I hoped they might have somebody who could also deal with facial injuries. However, I sadly and apprehensively felt that by the morning, in spite of the antibiotics (because the injury had happened so many hours previously), infection would have taken hold. I fully expected to find him with a fulminating meningitis the next day, and in no condition to travel at all.

I could not contain my amazement when I went to the ward first thing, and found him sitting by his bed while it was being made by the nurse, and apart from the fact that his was still sporting his arrow, he seemed not much the worse!

Just at that moment, we were told to stand by for the visit of the Minister of Health who had suddenly decided to do his own ward round. The great man proceeded slowly down the ward, politely greeting each patient. When he came to my man of the night before, he stopped and asked what had happened.

Well, said the patient, he had just been in the market when somebody had taken a pot-shot at him. No, he didn't know why.

I thought that the Minister would at least ask what could be done, and how the man felt, and other similar questions, or perhaps offer to find money to fund some transport to get the man to Kano quickly. But no. He thought for a minute and then asked, "Have they charged the man who did it?" And that was his only response. He passed on to the next bed.

The upshot of this story was that, our ambulance being out of action, the next available transport was the hospital Land Rover, itself in a very precarious condition. The Matron volunteered to travel with the patient in this vehicle, taking with her food, morphia, penicillin and a few other items deemed advisable. When she eventually returned to Maiduguri, she told us what a horrific journey they had had. Soon after setting off, the brakes half failed, and the 400 miles journey was completed with a more than dodgy braking system. Moreover, the driver flatly refused to keep going at prayer time, but insisted on stopping at intervals so that he could get out of the vehicle and pray appropriately (although he was a Moslem, I had been given to understand that he would have been excused his prayers on such a journey). Matron feared that they would never get there that day, or if they did it would not be before having an accident en route, but finally, and thankfully, they limped into Kano and she was able to decant her patient, surprisingly still surviving well, at the hospital there.

Some time later on, I contacted the surgeon in Kano to ask what had happened. He told me that they had managed to get the arrow out without doing any further damage; that the eyeball had not been involved at all, luckily; and that the wound had healed up cleanly straight away without any infection at all. The man had actually gone back to Potiskum within a few days, no long lasting harm done. I expect by the time I was enquiring he would have been back in his local market again – dodging further arrows?

An amusing tailpiece in connection with this case was that when the nurse first rang me to tell me that an emergency had arrived at the hospital, he had said to me, "Doctor, we have an emergency – it is an arrow shoot."

"You mean an arrow wound," I replied. "No," he told me, "It is an arrow shoot because the arrow is still there." So now we know.

In addition to the few of us who were Government employees, there were one or two Mission settlements in the general area. One, a few miles out of Maiduguri, was the Molai leprosy settlement with its own small hospital. I always enjoyed a visit there, driving along a rough bush road out of the station. I expect the Molai people would just as much enjoy a trip into Maiduguri where provisions could be bought. Compared with Molai we would be the 'bright light' centre. The Molai Mission staff were always thought of by the rest of us as being part of our expatriate community in Maiduguri, and indeed somebody always came in to Maiduguri from there on Sundays to take the Christian services which were held in the Courthouse on the GRA (Government Reservation Area – where the Senior Service staff lived). In later years, long after I had returned to the UK, we were told that permission to hold such services was withdrawn by the Nigerian authority (which had taken over with Independence), the general population being Moslem.

After I had developed my general routine, I had time to look around, and reflect on what I was seeing and doing. One thing which struck me very forcibly, though I think in retrospect that I was possibly making a rather harsh judgment, was that the Africans seemed to have little empathy with each other. Not much allowance was made for anyone who might be feeling pretty ill and perhaps in pain. This seemed to me to apply to the nursing staff as well as to the general populace. For instance, one evening a father came in to the hospital on his bicycle, followed by a young boy of perhaps ten years old. The father had indeed brought the child in for help – but had not carried him or wheeled him along on the bike saddle. The boy had a nasty penetrating wound of one eye and must have been in a lot of pain, yet he had to walk, even trot in order to keep up with Dad. There was concern here, and recognition that help was needed, but nothing, I thought, of compassion as I understood it.

The most extreme example of this happened when I was working in another station – Katsina. An adolescent girl crawled on her hands and knees in to the outpatient clinic one morning. She had patiently waited her turn among the fifty or so others who were squatting on the verandah outside. She looked to be in a very bad way, almost grey with pallor. She was clearly very anaemic, and the only thing to do was to get her straight on the ward and start investigations immediately so that I could begin to treat her urgently. We had nothing like blood transfusions, so 'quickly' would only just be quick enough if we were lucky. I took blood for testing while she was with me, sent it to our lab technician, and gave the nurse instructions to admit the child forthwith.

Some fifty or so patients later on, with the clinic finished, I left the surgery en route for the wards. Crawling again on hands and knees across the dusty compound, accompanied by a nurse, I saw the young girl, struggling to proceed. I had imagined her to be tucked up in bed an hour before.

"Whatever is she here in the compound for?" I asked the nurse.

"She is being admitted – I am taking her to the ward," was the surprised reply.

"This child is very seriously ill – you can see that she is too weak to walk," I said, "Go get a stretcher and somebody to help you – she is to be carried."

The nurse looked astonished – she simply did not understand my concern. However one of the labourers and a stretcher were found and we carried the poor child to her bed. Half an hour later, she died. The blood test had indicated anaemia so profound that it had not even been measurable. Why did none of the clinic nurses see how ill and weak she was? And if they did, why did they not act accordingly? Surely I was not the only person to realise what a desperately ill patient we had here.

The only explanation I can offer is that so often, especially in outlying areas, survival could be a struggle and life was therefore pretty cheap. There was no sense in wasting energy and effort on others that you might be wiser to conserve for yourself. Was I right? I didn't know. It was all difficult to work out.

Another thing which was endemic was, as I mentioned earlier on, the need to 'pay' for services. Patients would sometimes have to pay a nurse to bring a bedpan or a drink. They might have to 'pay' the *mai gardi* (the gateman) to be allowed into the hospital compound in the first place. This sort of thing didn't only happen within the hospital context. For instance, my cook-steward, Ali, (who had replaced Samuel), had a brother who was a trader in another town. From time to time he sent some money to Ali in the form of a postal order. Invariably Ali, when he received one of these remittances, asked me if I would cash it at the Post Office for him, because he knew that I would receive the full and correct amount, whereas he might only be given some of it, while the clerk kept some for himself as 'commission'. Expatriates, it seemed, were not treated like this. I was warned, however, when I first arrived, always to watch the cashier if I was withdrawing money at the bank, and count it myself as he flipped the notes through at the other side of the counter – a habit I have never subsequently rid myself of.

My husband, when he was Principal of a training college, was sometimes offered great wads of money by hopeful fathers who wanted their sons to be accepted as students. Needless to say he always declined this, saying that to do so was "not his custom" ('custom' was understandable – people respected that). The whole system depended on patronage it seemed sometimes – well, for 'patronage' read 'bribes'.

Yet there was a Kanuri woman who from time to time had come to see me in the clinic for various ailments. Although she occasionally brought me a few eggs, I am sure she never thought she was 'paying' me for the help she received – I think she genuinely meant 'thank you'. I never felt that she spoke to me as anything but an equal, and I don't think she ever felt the need to sweeten me up. In fact, when I left Maiduguri for Katsina in August 1958, and the hospital staff laid on a 'Send-off' party for me, she attended. This party was a formal affair, to which members of the public were able to come, and they were also allowed to speak when the agenda reached the item 'Free speeches'. I had not spotted her until the Free Speeches item arrived, and at that point she rose and said how much she had benefited by seeing me and that she wanted to thank me publicly so that everyone would know what I had done for her. For a woman to take a prominent role like that in an Islamic society at that time was amazing, I thought, and I was much touched by her gesture.

Chapter 10

On the social side of life in Maiduguri, to coin a phrase, I had never had it so good. In spite of being busy, I never lacked for invitations out to dinner, drinks parties, curry lunches (on Sundays), Club nights, the cinema and so on. Always controlled by the fact that when it was my week on call I had to be available for and contactable by the hospital, day or night, I nevertheless managed to have a pretty full life, and indeed, welcomed quiet evenings when I could stay home on my own.

Except for the rainy season we never saw clouds, so that even if there was no moon, the skies would always be brilliant with stars that sparkled like diamond-fire on black velvet. I have never forgotten the first time that I identified the Southern Cross, albeit a bit distorted as we were still a bit too far north of the equator for it to be, as one might say, straight up and down. It was a thrill to recognise something about which I had only ever read until then. The whine of the mosquitoes, the chirruping of the crickets and the ever present sound of bare feet padding on the sand only served to accentuate the absence of daytime noises when I was sitting out in the late evening. The sound of a snatch of conversation from the open windows and doors of somebody else's house not far away made you realise how quiet and tranquil it was in your own if you were having a peaceful evening all to yourself.

Once a month in the Maiduguri station, on a Saturday evening, we had what we called Open Night at the club. This was a social occasion when we had supper and dancing. Each month a different department organised the food, using an allowance of money from club funds for it. Generally, because most of the expatriate wives did not have jobs, it was they who had time to turn to and get everything ready. But in the Medical Department, except for Louis, a bachelor, we were all working women – me and the three nursing sisters. It was quite a job for us to fit everything in to what was a pretty normal working day for us. Luckily we all had good cooks, especially me. Ali was the envy of the whole station it sometimes seemed. People would say "It's not fair, she has the best cook on the station, and all she ever eats herself is a lettuce leaf!"

Ali proved his worth on Club Nights. I would have bought in what we needed from the canteens, and he would have come home from the market with chickens and ducks and rice and any other items he could get. He would start cooking soon after lunch, and later on he and I together would begin to make up the rest of my contribution to the buffet. We would work hard so that everything would be ready for the evening. Obviously one didn't get food ready too early in the heat. None of us had fridges that would cater for sixty or eighty. One time, though, when we had just started, I was called to the hospital for an emergency. Telling Ali that I would be back as soon as ever I could, I got into the car and dashed off. I just hoped he would be able to manage and that I wouldn't be too late delivering my contribution to the Club. I need not have worried. When I finally got back home, everything was ready, beautifully presented and there was nothing left for me to do. Ali was sitting quietly by the back door, imperturbable as usual, dressed in his spotless white uniform (you provided 'working dress' for the day time and 'evening uniform' for later, when the household chores were done, for all your boys). He really was wonderful and I was very lucky to have him working for me.

Everyone would dress up for Open Night – the men would wear dinner jackets or white monkey jackets (mostly the latter as they were cooler), and cummerbunds, and the women would put on either long evening gowns or their prettiest short cocktail dresses. I saved my best and rather expensive 'ball gown' (which I still have, though at my advanced age I can't get it on any more) for very special occasions like Christmas and New Year. However, before sailing for Nigeria I had made myself a simpler long cotton evening dress to be worn for more ordinary occasions. I still have that one too, and can still get it on comfortably, though as old ladies in their eighties don't expose their elderly arms and necks, it isn't worn any more! We would, on Open Nights, dance to records after the supper. More often than not we would go outside onto a large concrete square in the compound for the purpose, as it was so much cooler there. Dancing would continue for as long as there was anybody to carry on. I was generally so tired after a long hard week that, like Cinderella, I usually took myself home to bed at about midnight. But I always enjoyed Open Nights – they were fun.

Although Maiduguri was quite a big station as stations went, with sixty to eighty expatriates, perhaps rather more with the wives, we were like a big family rather than a village. Everybody soon knew everybody else, and on the whole we all pulled together well. We all worked hard, but we all knew how to relax and enjoy ourselves as well. This was important, for other than the tiny cinema (and in many if not in most stations there would not be such an amenity), and apart from our annual Agricultural Show, occasional race meetings and the very rare durbars, there were no other outside entertainments. We made our own amusements therefore, either at the Club or in our own houses. Everyone held dinner or lunch parties, usually at weekends rather than midweek, and one tried hard to find different topics for conversation, otherwise it was all too easy to use just what was happening in station for 'news' because there simply wasn't anything else. That could make things very gossipy, and not really very interesting. I took a weekly copy of the Sunday Observer so had items from there to talk about. Others would listen to the BBC World Service on their radios, so we did keep up with the rest of the world to some extent.

An invitation to dinner at the Residency was a bit like a royal command. As I have said, anyone new coming into the station was expected to sign the Resident's Book. In Maiduguri this was kept during the day in a huge dome-like edifice made out of woven grass which was sited at the gate to the Resident's compound and guarded by a Native Authority policeman, who would solemnly admit you to sign the book. The British Resident was the British Government representative and senior administrator for the whole province. He was really quite important, and had a Senior District Officer and various District Officers to support him, who, like the Resident himself, would spend a lot of time out on tour, visiting the various districts in the province, seeing the Nigerian District Heads and dealing with all sorts of things, from purely administrative duties to sorting out misdemeanours and other problems that the District Heads found to be beyond them.

Tom Letchworth was the Resident when I was there first, and he and his wife Marjorie were well loved and regarded by us all as the mother and father of the station. They had worked out a 'formula' for dinner parties. When you arrived, you would be shown into the lounge and offered sherry. There you would meet the other guests for the night – usually anything up to a dozen of us. After a suitable interval, Marjorie would 'collect' the women with her eye, and sweep us upstairs in order to freshen up (which meant 'Do you need to visit the loo before the meal?'). Tom meanwhile would 'collect' the men and take them elsewhere for the same purpose. The Residency was probably superior to most other Government houses, and I suppose had an extra loo. In nearly all the other houses, the women would be taken to the only bathroom, while the men, should they have the need, would go out into the compound to 'see Africa' as they delicately put it. No wonder all our bougainvillea and frangipani bloomed so profusely! After this interlude, we were conducted into the dining room where, in the Maiduguri Residency, there was a splendid huge round table. A very nice meal would be served, with so many courses that I almost lost count, always ending with a savoury before coffee. We would sit there drinking our coffee for quite a long time, and talking, and then finally the Resident and his wife would rise and go to the doorway, through which we would all file, shaking hands with them and thanking them before leaving. It was a neat way, I always thought, of being hospitable without hurrying people, and yet ensuring that the evening was brought to a tidy end at a reasonable hour. I always enjoyed dinner at the Residency when Tom and Marjorie were there. They were such nice people.

When they heard the news of my engagement some months later, they immediately invited me to be married from the Residency, and indeed had me to stay with them for the last week before the wedding, for I would have to vacate my house and would normally have booked in at the Rest House. I was very grateful to them both. They looked after me like a daughter, and Marjorie went to a great deal of trouble to find flowers for a bouquet for me on 'the day', and also to arrange the reception, which they also hosted from the Residency. They gave us a wonderful send-off and I have never forgotten their kindness. But more of that later on in this saga.

I have mentioned the race meetings in Maiduguri. They were held quite frequently, and were like no race meetings I had ever seen in England! For a start, the course itself was just soft sand – no grass. It was fenced off as in the UK, but that was all. There was no hope of really seeing how things were progressing in a race even if you had binoculars – and I hadn't any anyway. All you could do was to watch the cloud of dust thrown up by the galloping horses as it moved round the course. You could sometimes see the leading horse. How any of the jockeys except the one riding the foremost animal could see what was happening or how they were doing I never knew, for they must all have been half blinded by the flying sand. I remember that in Maiduguri there was one particular white horse which ran in just about every race on the card, right through the afternoon – and when it ran, it always won, so the bets, I suppose, would be more for the second and third places, for the first was always pre-ordained, or so it seemed.

The saddling enclosure was a small sandy area just behind the Tote. Here the horses were tethered, some lucky ones in a spot of shade, and the others in the blazing sun. All were open to anything and anyone, and not protected from the public in any way. The saddles were ordinary everyday saddles. I saw nothing remotely resembling racing saddles as I had seen them in the UK. The jockeys too, didn't appear to have racing silks or even special colours – they just wore ordinary trousers, or Moslem ones, and shirt tops. Most wore the ordinary 'hula' or embroidered cap that men wore there – no proper jockey's caps, or very few. The weighing in scales were set up outside on the sand, but although all jockeys had to be weighed, I noticed that there seemed to be no restriction on their having drinks – Fanta Orange, Krola (an African kind of coca cola), or anything else after having weighed in.

A constant group of youths was always in the saddling enclosure, intent on stealing what they could. The ploy was for them to get together and start to run round and round in circles, surrounding one or more of the riders. They would run faster and faster, causing total confusion, in the midst of which one of them would dart in and snatch anything he could – a cap, a whip, anything. By the time the others had slowed down, the young thief was out and away and nobody could then catch him. Slick work!

We had a Tote, and this was always staffed by the Europeans, for the locals did not trust each other. I sometimes spent hours in the Tote, not understanding at all what the terms meant, but I could at least sell tickets and I learnt which ones to sell for what requests. I was also asked a few times to be the Assistant Starter, sharing the honours with the Official Starter who was at that time one of the senior Agricultural Officers, Mallam Lawan, an extremely nice and courteous man.

One thing which made race days very popular with the Africans was that they were then allowed to gamble, but only within the race-course grounds. This didn't mean just betting on the horses – it also meant that they could play cards or dice. So around the course, taking no notice at all of the racing, would be groups of men playing cards and so on. Normally this was not allowed, but on race days...

Talking of gambling, if you went to the cinema (and as it was outdoor, films could only be shown at night when it was dark, by the way), you would often see groups of men sitting on the benches there, not watching the film at all, but playing cards in the light shining from the screen, knowing full well that to do so was really forbidden.

However, when the proper lights went on, say between an A and a B film, the cards would be scooped away in a second in case any police were standing in the cinema to pounce on gamblers.

Yes, race days were fun and I always enjoyed them. There was a sort of stand erected for spectators, but it looked rather shaky to me and when everyone got excited as the cloud of dust which was the group of runners approached the finishing post, I used to think that the whole thing would collapse and that within moments I would be called away to receive casualties at the hospital along the road. Fortunately this never happened. Louis was not interested in racing or riding at all, so he, bless him, always offered to be on call on race days so that I could indulge my 'vice'.

Chapter 11

Government medical officers were not normally allowed to attend any patients on a private basis – we had to confine our duties to Government service as one would expect. However, in some outlying stations where there was no other doctor, and Maiduguri was one of these, Government doctors were allowed to see an occasional patient privately so long as this did not interfere with the duties for which they were officially employed. I was asked to see private patients only a handful of times in all the years I was out in Nigeria. Once I was asked to see an Arab lady at her home – she was in very strict purdah even there, and wore a veil over the whole of her face when I saw her. The first time I saw her I was able to treat her at home, but some time later when I was asked to see her again, I managed to persuade her husband to allow her to be admitted to the hospital for a short time. The reason for that was that I was about to go out on tour, and I knew that Louis would have quite enough on his plate looking after the whole hospital on his own, without having to go out to do domiciliary visits. This lady was quite ill and needed a good deal of monitoring. I was pleased when she came to the ward, as I felt it showed trust in us, and that was important to Louis and me. The more we were trusted, the more we knew that word would get round, and hopefully that meant that more people would come to us for help in good time instead of waiting until the last minute.

I always found it difficult to quote a fee and to accept payment when seeing patients in their own homes, for I felt that I was being adequately paid by Government for what I did. At the same time, I realised that if I did not stipulate a fee, many other people would expect home visits – people who would normally have come to the outpatient clinics. This sort of thing was like trying to cut the heads of the hydra – it could be never ending, and after all, we were there to see to the hospital and the Province, and not spend our time trotting round the town. However, those whom I did see at home could never understand it when I was hesitant about naming my fee. One husband who had asked me to go to his house to see his children, who were not well, asked me how much he owed me.

"Well, nothing really," was my reply, "I am paid by the Government."

"Nonsense!" he said, "There has to be a fee. Tell me what it is."

Reluctantly I suggested a few shillings.

"Not enough!' he snapped. "Say again."

I added a shilling or two to my initial suggestion.

"Not enough!" was his further reply, "You must take more!"

I stood my ground, however, and finally got away, but not before explaining that as a Government Medical Officer, whether I took a fee or not made no difference to the attention I gave – I would always do my best for whoever I saw. To do otherwise would not be my way. Being a businessman, with an eye to charging for services rendered, I think he thought I was quite mad, but as he never hesitated to ask me to visit if he was worried about his family, and always insisted on paying me, perhaps he thought that even if I was crazy, I was reliable.

During the course of a day, the unexpected often happened, though generally at the hospital. One did not anticipate the unusual around one's own house before breakfast, though. But one morning, before I had left the house to go down to the hospital, I was called by my steward to speak to the steward of a family whose compound was near mine. This neighbouring steward had come to ask my help because his wife had given birth to a premature baby. I grabbed a pair of scissors and went tearing across the compounds to find the young wife sitting on a mat in the corner of a rather bare concrete floored room, laughing at us all as though she found the whole situation amusing. Probably she was really rather embarrassed. Her tiny little baby had been carefully laid on the floor, and covered with a few none too clean wrappings. It was still attached to the placenta which had also been delivered. Her husband found some string, and we boiled it and my scissors for ten minutes in a kettle, and then I tied off and cut the cord, and got both mother and baby down to the maternity ward for supervision for a couple of days. I am happy to say that both did well and soon returned home.

Many people, I found, thought that wherever and whenever they could waylay you – in the office, halfway across the hospital compound, even in your own house, you would stop and examine and treat them, even though they well knew the hospital procedure. Everyone wanted favours and many would try to bribe you. Happily, as mentioned earlier, everyone respected 'custom' so when you politely refused the offer, explaining why, your refusal was accepted.

A lot of people seemed to think that it was advisable to get a letter written to hand to you, in which they described their symptoms and requests for medicine. Sometimes people wrote themselves, while others paid local scribes to do it for them. No women ever wrote, but a number of Southern Nigerian men brought letters to me in which they had set out various and often bizarre symptoms suffered by their wives, finishing with requests for diagnoses on the basis of the letters. These letters were often very amusing to read, though I must make it clear straight away that I did not 'laugh' at them for I knew they were sent in all seriousness. Once I mentally translated them into my own idiomatic English, I knew what they meant. Everyone did their best, and it depended on how much English they had at their command. And who was I to put them down? I didn't have a full command of Hausa, and only a very few words in Kanuri. Many a time I think the nurses who interpreted for me and the patients must have had a good laugh at my own inept attempts to get down to the basics in a language not my own. I often had to resort to mime – and if you can consider miming the complaints, for instance, of acute diarrhoea, or of 'fever and pains all over' (the ubiquitous description of malaria), you will see what I mean. It was essential to keep one's sense of humour – mutual laughter is a great leveller. If you couldn't laugh you might as well pack up and go back to England I always thought – but laughter had not to be in any way hurtful. It was important too to be able to laugh at yourself. The old adage 'laugh and the world laughs with you' applied here absolutely.

There was always so much to do, and I often felt, and told my family back home in the UK, that it was like trying to repair a collapsing wall when bricks were falling off faster than they could be replaced. One never seemed to be able to catch up completely. I think the outpatient clinics were usually the busiest places. Often, when you thought you had finally cleared morning's work and that you could go home for lunch and hopefully a siesta, a message would come to say that another so many patients had arrived at outpatients and that even with the nurse filtering out those he or she could deal with, a great number were still waiting for you. You had to start all over again and clear the clinic once more. After having worked solidly in the heat since 7 o'clock in the morning until 2 p.m., which often included a stint in theatre and a 'surgery' at the Nursing Home, you would be more than ready to take a break, and although I loved what I was doing, there were moments like that when things were a tad daunting. Still, it all had to be done, and done it was. It was not unheard of to see a hundred patients in one morning's outpatient clinic, and then after that was the ward work – and theatre – and anything else that happened along.

As I said earlier, I had felt at first that people showed little compassion for each other. Perhaps this was indeed so, but I had also learnt that in a context where survival was paramount, there was often little room for sympathy or self sacrifice. It is important to add that I saw fellow feeling as well. Mothers would stay in hospital with their children, bring food for them, and fan them to keep the flies off their faces. Similarly, people would also come to bring food for adult friends or family members, and in turn would stay during the day, waving huge fans over them to keep them cool and comfortable. It should not be forgotten either, that efforts would be made to bring sick or injured people to the hospital, sometimes over great distances, using whatever transport was available – oxcarts, bicycles, donkeys and so on.

There was some degree of protocol about this as well. If a 'big' man – i.e. somebody important, was admitted, then there would always be several minions sitting around his bed, attending to him. You didn't see this on the women's ward usually, as women were not so important! Only once did I see this sort of thing happen, and that was in the Senior Service Nursing Home, where we once had a young Kanuri woman admitted, the wife of an African Senior Service officer. She had never been in hospital before. Several women of her household arrived with her, and settled themselves down in her room, squatting on the floor around her bed. At the end of the day, to my consternation, they all began to unroll sleeping mats, clearly preparing to stay the night with her. I expostulated, saying that now it was night, they should go home and let her rest. They would be able to return in the morning, I told them. They said that she must not be left alone. I told them that there would be somebody on duty all night, so that she would not be left. "But," they said, "she is not used to being alone at night – we always sleep in the same room. She will be afraid without us." The young woman confirmed this. It seemed that she had never been on her own in a room at night, and she was genuinely afraid of the solitude. I compromised in the end and allowed two people to stay. The others reluctantly departed. This was where understanding and sympathy were clearly shown. Nigeria was often a country of paradoxes.

In some areas of Northern Nigeria, I was told, Islamic law still prevailed and I heard of thieves who had a hand cut off as punishment. This probably happened in outlying areas, as I never actually saw that for myself. In Maiduguri we had an Alkali's Court. The Alkali (pronounced al-kar-lee) was a Native Authority judge or magistrate. We also had a prison. One of the duties of the medical officer was to examine prisoners regularly to see if they were fit to receive punishment. This usually consisted of so many lashes with the *bulala*, or whip. We also had to see any men accused of murder, to decide if they were fit to plead before they were tried. Sometimes if young boys had been taken into custody, we were asked to say how old they were – presumably because they had to be of a certain age before they could be tried in court, or given certain punishments. It was always difficult to estimate an age for anyone. We simply had to guess at their ages – children mature at different times, there would be those who had not been particularly well nourished and who would be undersized, and there would be those who had some sort of chronic condition – recurrent malaria, hookworm, schistosomiasis, whatever, and these could all affect growth and development, and therefore general appearance. We simply had to make educated guesses, taking into consideration the general appearance of the child or youth. Although it was possible to register non-native births, there was no generalised system of birth certification in Northern Nigeria at that time. One way of determining age was to ask the individual concerned if they remembered various incidents – for instance if he remembered the visit of a certain VIP, or any other big event which had happened in the previous few years – something which could help to pinpoint the time of his birth.

Back to the local prisons and our examining those accused of murder. Several of these people had been languishing in prison for many months, even years, because witnesses had fled to bush, being afraid of appearing in court. Some of the accused would say to me that they were willing to plead guilty in order to have their cases tried and done with – indeed some even told me that they had pleaded guilty a long time ago, so as to get everything over, but that they were simply told they must let the system take its course. They were very despondent. It was the captivity that they hated, not the idea of official punishment.

When somebody had been sentenced to a flogging, he would be brought to the hospital, handcuffed to a warder, with a note saying that he had been sentenced to, say, fifty lashes, or a hundred, or whatever it might be – and was he fit to receive them? What do you do? I would examine the man and ask him a few questions about his general health, after which I had to make my decision. I didn't like the idea of flogging, though I knew that in fact it was often done quite lightly – more as a means of humiliation than anything. Moreover, this was a mandatory and official punishment, laid down by the Native Authority, so it had to be complied with. I could not say that a healthy man was unfit, therefore. However, it was within my power to recommend fewer lashes than had been decided upon, and on occasions that is what I did if I felt that the total number laid down was excessive. Occasionally I found that the culprit really wasn't a very healthy specimen, and then I could honestly – and thankfully – say that he was not fit.

One had to remember that lashes were always open to abuse, and we knew that from time to time there would be somebody who would take advantage of the sentence and administer punishment very harshly. It was not easy to make a medical decision, and you had to try to set aside your own personal feelings as much as possible, and be impartial. It was the local law and it was not for the medical officer to undermine it. I am glad to say that any man who had marks on his back after a beating was quickly brought to the hospital to be seen by the medical officer, and should we have thought that things had got out of hand, we were able to take action to put a stop to, shall I say, over-exuberance.

An example of estimating ages by the timing of events came to my notice in a wholly different context, and was in respect of an older man. Shortly

84

after I arrived in Maiduguri, realising that the sooner I spoke some Hausa the better, I had arranged to have Hausa lessons. My teacher was a local man, Mallam Birma, and he came to my house each week for my lesson. In the course of conversation he told me a bit about himself. He had been born in a village in Biu Province, many miles from Maiduguri. When he was still a baby, the villagers learnt that a 'Mistereebee', an Englishman, was coming. It was said that he was going to build a road from Maiduguri to Biu. Everyone in the village was afraid of this 'Mistereebee', being convinced that he would kill and eat them. So en masse they fled into the bush where they lived for many months, living off the land and keeping well hidden. Mallam Birma said, "It was the rainy season for a lot of that time, and everyone got very wet and cold – all except for me. I was a very tiny baby, so my mother put me in a big calabash, which she covered and she carried me about in it. To this day," he went on, "my friends and family still call me 'The Calabash Baby'." 'Mistereebee', he told me, was in fact Mr Hewby, and he had indeed built the road to Biu, along which I was to drive when on tour a few months later. By working things out, I realised that my tutor, Mallam Birma, would be in his fifties, as indeed he looked to be. It was interesting to me then to note that my house in Maiduguri was on Hewby Avenue. Mr Hewby was also the first British Resident in Bornu. He would have been Resident in the early 1900s, which again would fit in well with the age I had estimated for Mallam Birma.

I mentioned the prisoners. From time to time a prisoner would be admitted to the hospital, and when this happened, he was always shackled to his bed, and a warder always accompanied him. Should the prisoner need the latrine, the warder would be there to unshackle him and go with him to the loo, and then reattach him to his bed afterwards. I think it was always a nice little rest for the warders, for they would just sit about on the verandahs while their charges were patients. Funnily enough on the other hand, we relied on prisoner labour for the cutting of the grass in the hospital compound. A small gang of them would be escorted to the hospital by one, maybe two, warders. The warders would then sit in the shade, perhaps dozing, for an hour or two, while the prisoners wielded their machetes, hacking away at the coarse and somewhat sparse grass. No prisoners to my knowledge ever tried to abscond. They all worked through the morning before being led away back to the prison at the end of their stint. I rather think that some of the prisoners were possibly more comfortable and better fed in prison than out of it.

Once or twice I had to go to the prison building itself – where the men were held literally behind bars. There were buildings where they could go inside, but these opened to the compound, where most of the men would spend the day before being locked in at night. However, the area was bounded by strong mesh so that nobody could escape. I would be conducted into a small anteroom where, if I had to see any prisoner, he would be brought to me there. There were a few women being held as well, and they had a separate but similar area cheek by jowl with that for the men.

When I was out on tour in Biu, I was asked to visit the prison there. This was different from that in Maiduguri, consisting of several long low breeze block buildings, rather like hospital wards in shape and size. They were in fact dormitories, and the prisoners were locked in them at night, but were out working during the day. Biu prison compound was spotlessly clean, and much smaller than the one in Maiduguri. At the time of my visit, which was in the morning, there were no prisoners on site. They were all out on various working parties. I imagine that they did tasks like repairing roads, which probably meant sweeping sandy surfaces to a reasonably level state after heavy lorries carrying cotton or groundnuts had churned things into deep ruts.

Chapter 12

Now, all these years on, I realise that I have almost forgotten what the extreme heat felt like. If my father had not kept just about every letter that I sent, I don't think I would now have recalled it properly. These letters mention the heat from time to time. I tell my parents that I generally had to change my clothes three times every 24 hours, because almost before I had put them on they were soaked with sweat. I point out how much more so this state of affairs is when we were operating because then we also had to wear rubber aprons, caps, gowns and masks, and rubber gloves. We were positively dripping when a theatre session ended, even though in Maiduguri we usually did our theatre sessions at 7 a.m. before the day really hotted up. In Katsina, another station I went to, I don't remember it being quite so hot, but as it was much nearer the edge of the Sahara desert, that surprises me now. Perhaps I had acclimatised even more by that time – or perhaps we had a better fan in the theatre there. There was no air conditioning in either place, just the fan over the table.

I found that in the extreme heat, and also when it was both hot and humid just before the rains, I used to get some prickly heat – that was a sort of rash which both itched and was sore as well. As soon as the Harmattan started, and it was minimally cooler – and when the humidity in the air went down to nil – then all the prickly heat disappeared. However, one's skin then became very dry. During Harmattan my heels would crack and bleed, as did my fingertips, just like they do here in the UK in very cold weather when it is frosty. When the humidity was high, my hair was always damp and I used to say that it smelt all the time of wet laundry! In the dry season it was dull and wispy. One way and another it never looked really nice!

An amusing aspect to the dry season, which lasted in Maiduguri for nine months of the year, was that there was so much static electricity about that I seemed to strike sparks off everything I touched – the car door, or a pile of clean clothes just after they had been ironed being two examples. After I was married, my husband and I were always highly amused to see – and feel (rather painfully I have to say) – a spark pass between our lips as we kissed each other before going off to our separate places of work in the morning. The sparks crackled too, quite loudly. Later on when the children were born, I would get sparks and a slight shock from them as well.

In the far north of Nigeria, the air humidity was always low or non-existent, except, as I said, just before the rains. This meant that at least one's laundry dried within a very short time of being hung out. Sometimes only minutes were enough. To illustrate the speed of drying, I have a good tale to tell... We had a carpet in our lounge that my husband had bought several years before we met. It was, I suppose, about twelve feet square. I decided that after so many years of dusty Harmattans it would be a good idea to shampoo it. In due course I managed to buy a bottle of carpet shampoo, and I told our boys that as soon as I had time I would show them how it was used and we would do this carpet.

I was rather busy for the next week or two however, and in the end my small boy must have decided that I'd forgotten. At all events, he decided, unknown to me, that he would take matters into his own hands. When I arrived home that lunch time, I found that he had emptied the whole bottle of carpet shampoo into the bath – the bath being full of the water that we were keeping there for general use in case the regular supply was cut off, as it often was. Having stirred up a great lather, he had then lifted the carpet, and had plunged it somehow into the bath where he had given it a good rub-a-dub, just as he did the ordinary household washing. He told me that it had not been easy to do as the carpet was so big! However, he assured me that he had washed and rinsed it well. He was just trying to wring it out as I arrived home. Wring out a carpet? Impossible of course. So, we heaved it, dripping wet, out of the bath and into the compound, where we draped it over all our small occasional tables so that it (hopefully) would not pick up sand as it certainly would do if we laid it on the ground. Twenty minutes later it was bone dry and we put it back on the lounge floor. How's that for speed? I have to say it looked very bright and clean.

One very quickly adapted to the heat. I wrote in one of my early letters home that I thought Harmattan must be on the way because I had suddenly felt so cold one morning that I had put on a cardigan. I laughed heartily at myself for doing that when I looked at the thermometer and found that the temperature had indeed dropped – to 80 degrees Fahrenheit – and I was feeling cold! I had been in Maiduguri for just six weeks. Generally the heat was such that when I went to crash out on my bed for a siesta, the sheets and pillows felt quite hot to the touch, and when I went to the wardrobe to get a clean dry dress, all the clothes inside also felt as hot to touch as if they had just been ironed. Yet after a time you didn't think this strange – in fact you hardly noticed. Because the water supply tanks were in the roof space, they also got very hot, so that the 'cold' water often came out of the taps too hot to use immediately. The roofs in many houses were made of corrugated metal, which heated up tremendously.

In the hot season, which for us was from about the end of February to June when the rains started, we would – most of us anyway – put our beds

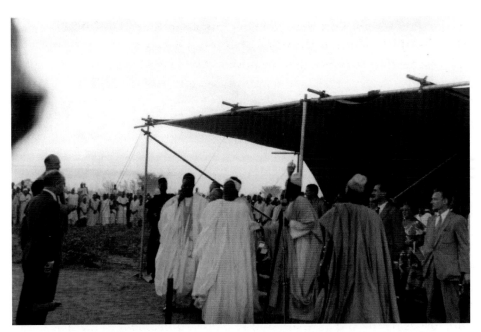

Beneath the canopy in white robes are Shettima Kashim Ibrahim, then Waziri of Bornu (left), and the Shehu of Bornu (right), 1957. The Shehu has just hammered in the short stake in front of him to mark the site of the future train station in Maiduguri at the end of the planned Bornu railway.

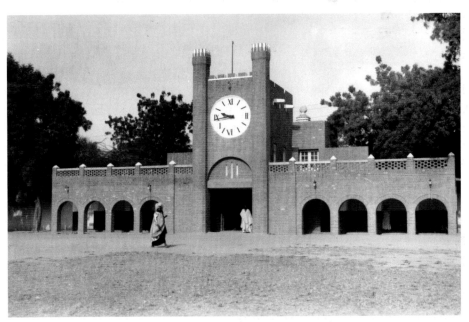

The Shehu's Palace, Maiduguri.

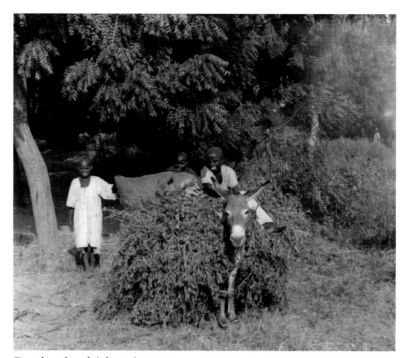

Donkey load (above).

Head load (below).

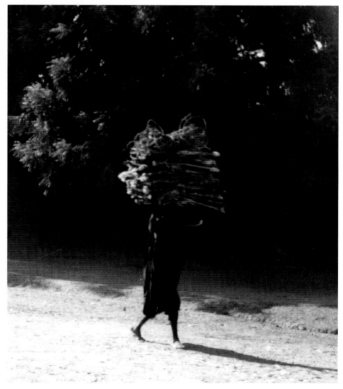

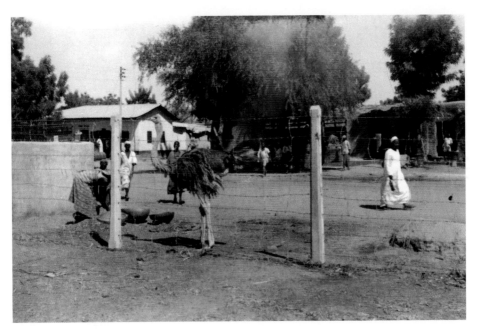

Maiduguri street scene.

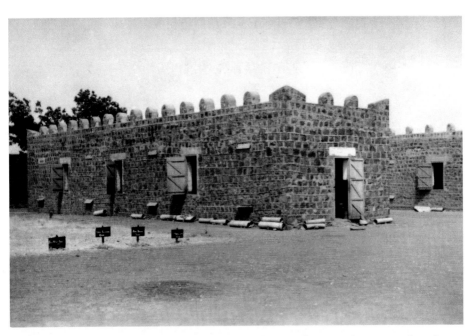

Biu Prison compound and dormitories. The markers in the ground indicate where men from each dormitory lined up for working parties.

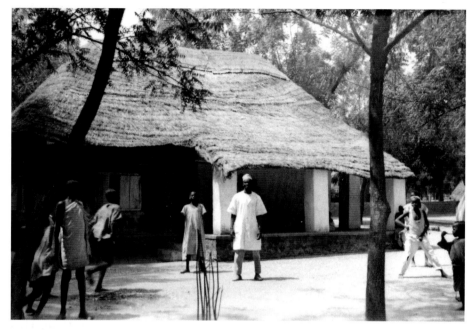

Shani Dispensary (Biu Division) with dispensary attendant and patients.

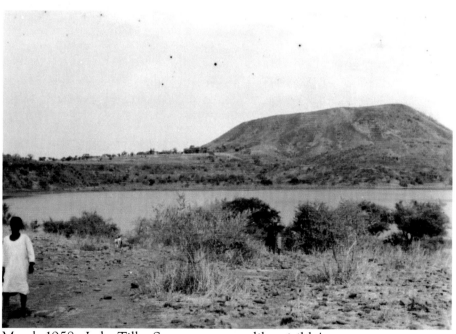

March 1958 - Lake Tilla. Sorry - no crocodiles visible!

outside into the compound because it was so hot inside. Many houses had special little sleeping-out areas bounded by shrubs for privacy. Our last house had two walled compounds, and we would put our beds out into the one at the back of the house. The children's beds came out too, onto the verandah, and we all slept outside. It still felt hot though – to such an extent even outside that we slept stark naked, with only the mosquito net between us and the sky. We always had to be sure that we woke in good time in the morning, so that we could be up and inside the house dressing by the time our boys unlocked the compound door and came on duty. But sleeping out under the stars was really very nice.

The Hot Season was followed by the Rainy Season. The rains were preceded by a few weeks when it was still very hot indeed but also extremely humid – you knew that the rains were on the way and wished that they would come soon to relieve the heat. The humidity made for a lot of prickly heat rashes, even in the Africans themselves. I can remember one African patient coming to see me at the Nursing Home clinic because he had so much prickly heat – and it was so bad that he did not sit down for the consultation but stood up against the door frame, scratching his back against it the whole time. This rash could be really very distressing.

Africa is the only place I have ever lived in where one could actually smell rain that had fallen many miles away. We would sometimes, at that time of the year, feel our hearts lifting because the smell of rain was so pronounced. One would think 'Great! It must have been somewhere round about – we may have a downpour here today – or tomorrow – or...' only to have our hopes dashed by hearing later in the day that the rain had been at least fifty miles away. During this pre-rains time we could and did have dust storms, which were very uncomfortable. One often saw the dust devils whirling across the bush then. Once, some years after I was married and we had our two children, we had enjoyed a few days' local leave in Jos, 400 miles down the road. We were returning home by car, when, with a few miles still to go before we reached Maiduguri, we were hit by a massive dust storm. I had to pull in off the side of the road and park on the edge of the bush, and we shut all the car windows. It was stifling inside the car that way, but we had to endure it or we would have been half asphyxiated by the thick dust blowing against us. Visibility was absolutely nil – all that could be seen was the thick sandy dust against the windows. Nobody could have even walked through that. All sense of direction went and all you knew was that you were in the middle of this thick gritty maelstrom. The only thing to do was to wait. When it finally passed over us, the car was covered with it. A good deal had managed to filter inside in spite of the closed windows, and there was even more under the bonnet all over the engine – although because of driving over sand most of the time anyway, engines were always gritty and sandy even in the best of conditions. A bit more now and again didn't make much difference to the cars. We were very glad on this occasion to be able to open the windows and resume our journey, even if the outside atmosphere was still hot. At least now we had a draught going over us as we moved onwards. Once the dust storm had passed it was as if it had never happened. The sky was as clear as ever and the wind had subsided. For a long time afterwards my little daughter sang, "I don't like dust storms, I do like rain storms!"

Finally and thankfully, the rains would break. There would be a day when suddenly and unexpectedly the heavens would open and down would come the deluge. It would stop as suddenly, leaving wet sand underfoot, and there would be the lovely smell of wet dust, wet foliage, wet air, wet everything – and some degree of coolness too for a short time. I enjoyed the first time I experienced the rains. We had had that first sudden downpour during siesta that day. Some friends of mine laughed at themselves because they had been on their beds resting during the afternoon when they heard the rain. "We were so thrilled," they told me, "that we leapt off our beds and dashed out into the compound and danced around in the torrential rain. It was quite a few minutes before we realised that we had shot out stark naked as it had been so hot and sticky when we started our siesta. We hurried back in rather shamefacedly to put some clothes on!"

When I say 'torrential' I really do mean that. You would expect that our rain would soak straight through the sand in seconds – and yes, it did soak in, but amazingly there was just so much of it all at once that it took quite some time to disappear. I was driving down from my house to the hospital one morning when I was overtaken by a sudden heavy storm. On arrival, getting out of the car, I found that I had stepped into water which came well over my ankles – the hospital compound was like a sea. Half an hour later when I came off the ward, the water might never have been there at all – it had all gone into the sand. And my sandals were quite dry again too. The force of the rain, increased by the accompanying wind, could be considerable, as the following two anecdotes will show.

We happened at one time to have a round hole in one of the lounge windows. My small boy had somehow managed to puncture the window with the end of a broom handle. (I should have known better than to give him a proper broom when he was more accustomed to using the local 'broom' which was really a hand held bundle of twigs.) I knew this day that we were in for a storm, as a black menacing cloud was coming across the sky, but I was totally unprepared for what happened next. What happened next was that as the storm broke, a powerful jet of water, just like that from a fireman's hose at full pressure, burst through the hole in the window and shot about eighteen feet across the whole width of the room. It came in a completely horizontal line, and in seconds the whole room was flooded. There was nothing at all that any of us could do but wait until the rain stopped. Only then could we begin to mop up. I never saw anything like it before or since.

The second story showing the power of our storms was for me very frightening. Our garage at the time was built of breeze blocks, was quite roomy and pretty high. It had walls on three sides, and the fourth side was not built up at all, but had two tall wooden gates which opened outwards. They were built a bit on the style of five barred gates, with broad strips of wood fitted horizontally into the main frame, but they were very tall and also very heavy as I was to discover. I had just come back to the house, and had driven my car straight into the garage, both gates being propped open with strong sturdy poles as usual. I could see that a dust storm was building up some distance away across the bush and travelling quite quickly in my direction. As I turned to make for the house, the storm hit. There was, astonishingly, almost no dust, but the wind was so strong that it tore one of the garage gates completely off its hinges except for one remaining screw. I somehow managed to catch hold of it before it fell on me, and I simply did not dare to leave go because I realised that if it was whirled onto me by the wind I could have been badly hurt. In another couple of seconds the rain struck. Desperately I hung on to the huge gate, trying to prevent it from twisting and being hurled all over the car or injuring me. I shrieked for my houseboys who would, I knew, have come to help, but the noise of the wind and rain were such that I could hardly hear my own cries. Water was being forced into my mouth, nose, ears and eyes and I could hardly breathe.

How I managed to hold that gate I shall never know, but I managed to do so for the next twenty minutes, fearing all the time that I'd have to let it go. Eventually the storm subsided and I dragged the gate to the wall and managed to prop it up before going into the house in a state of total exhaustion and feeling half drowned. Not an experience I'd like to repeat. It took three of us to carry the gate to where it could be safely left until such time as it could be repaired.

We also had lots of tropical thunderstorms – dramatic, violent and utterly exhilarating. The whole atmosphere seemed to come alive then, and the lightning was often so vivid and continuous that at night, during a storm, it would rival the unrelenting brilliance of the noonday sun. An accompaniment to the rains was an army of frogs – or toads. One once got into the lounge and took refuge underneath a small set of bookshelves. The front of the shelves came down onto the floor, but at the back the bottom was open so that a small animal could hide there. This meant that the whole piece of furniture acted like a sounding box whenever the frog croaked, which seemed to be all the time. Our small boy was very cross with the frog and took it outside, dropping it onto the garden. Well, it wasn't long before another came in – and Momso once again removed the offending creature. I think he must have thought that there was only one frog in the whole of Maiduguri, for one day he said to me indignantly "Madam, yesterday I took that frog right down to the big road (this was some distance from the house) – and today it has come back again!"

After the rains we had what everyone called 'The Little Hot Season' – when it once again got pretty hot. That was the time of year when I first arrived. And following that we had our winter – Harmattan, the dry season. This was when the weather did get cooler and there was no humidity at all and one's skin got very dry as mentioned earlier. To combat this, I used what hand cream I could find – if indeed I could find any. In the end I found that Johnson's Baby Cream was better than anything else and I could usually find some of that in local shops.

During this time of the year a constant wind which brought dust from the Sahara, and therefore during these months there would be a thin layer of dust all over everything. No amount of dusting by the houseboys got rid of it – as fast as they worked, back it came. This was the time when the medical officers would do their touring, for some of the villages we had to visit were very remote, with occasionally no real roads to them. The only way to reach these places was to travel along dry riverbeds, so the driest season was obviously the one for us to choose. Moreover, the 'proper' roads were no longer washed out and closed because of the rain, so that even if they were rather rough, they were useable. The disadvantage of touring during Harmattan, however, was that because the atmosphere was so dusty, you couldn't take many decent photographs as everything was hazy. I was disappointed by that because I had hoped to get lots of pictures both to remember for myself and also to send home for my parents to see. Grand scenery just didn't present itself for me when I was out amongst it.

In my letters home, during November 1957 – my first November overseas – I told my parents about the many traders who came round the GRA to see what they could sell to the Europeans and other foreigners. They sold local craft work usually – lots of it I suppose was cheapjack stuff – but for newcomers like me it was all exotic. Moreover, with Christmas ahead, I was buying Christmas gifts for people back home, and what better than bits of exotica? I bought leather toys – a camel, a cow, for children in the family. I bought a leather handbag for my mother. I bought leather covers that could be stuffed and used as footstools, one of which I bought for my father. The leather was dyed with very bright colours (though one found in the end that the dye was actually not long lasting and faded a lot after several months).

There were small ivory objects – a bangle, a necklace, small carved animals. There were metal objects – anklets as worn by the Kanuri women, containers for the black eye make-up that they used. There were brass ornaments made in the likeness of various animals. There were knives, flywhisks, spearheads, and the brightly coloured feather fans of all sizes, used for keeping cool and also for keeping flies away. There were copper objects, wooden carvings, beads, all sorts. Everything imaginable was to be found in the traders' packs, or so it seemed. Already in November I was packing these gifts and posting them off by sea mail, for to send them all by airmail would have been quite expensive. I packed them all first in plastic bags before wrapping them up in brown paper, and I see from my letters that I asked my mother to return the bags because they were impossible to get hold of where I was, and they were very useful.

I also tried to get hold of Christmas cards. The only place where we could get stationery of any kind was a small Mission shop in the canteen area – known to us all as 'The Bookshop' where they sold writing paper, stationery of as many kinds as they could obtain, fancy goods, and so on. True to the spirit of Africa, their stock of Christmas cards had arrived – but with no matching envelopes! I bought just whatever envelopes they had that would do for my cards – some of which winged their way to England in huge foolscap sized ones. It was there that I found a box of twelve tiny baubles and a tiny little artificial Christmas tree – the last one in the shop. The little tree was all of a foot high with about half a dozen fold-out branches and the baubles were each less than an inch across. Now, more than fifty years on, only three of those little baubles remain and they are always the first to be put on my Christmas tree each year. They bring back so many memories and transport me straight into the heat and sun of Maiduguri every time. I shall be very sad when they finally disintegrate.

I told my family at this time, in my letter of 11th November 1957, just how hot it was, commenting that on the whole it was not all that terribly trying, only sometimes. I went on to say that in my bedroom, on the day that I was writing to them, with open windows and closed curtains and the fan going full pelt, my thermometer told me that it was 92 degrees Fahrenheit. I said that it was hotter outside, and that come the following March and the start of the Hot Season, it would be much more than that. It was, too.

Although it might seem sometimes that life was one long social whirl, I was working really very hard. I noticed that some illnesses predominated at different times of the year. For instance, in the rainy season we had a lot of cases of pneumonia – and also quite a number of minor fractures. The reason for the fractures? It was because sometimes, when the rains were very heavy, some of the mud houses began to collapse with the wet. If part of your house suddenly fell on you, then you could finish up with the odd broken bone. In the later part of the year we always anticipated an epidemic of meningitis, to such an extent that the Health Department sent supplies of sulphonamides round the province to the outlying dispensaries for general (controlled) distribution, to try to prevent any spread of infection, or indeed to try to prevent infection at all. This time of the year was very dry, and the Harmattan wind was starting up.

Accidents that we don't see in England were always happening here in Maiduguri. Somebody or other was always turning up with an arrow wound, for instance, because many people still used bows and arrows. One night, rather late, when I was just thinking of turning in, the phone rang.

"Doctor, can you come down?" asked the charge nurse, "We have a woman here who has been wounded by a spear."

A spear? At eleven o'clock at night? OK, I unlocked the door and got into my car again. It knew its way to the hospital all by itself, I thought, by now. Sure enough, there was a woman sitting there and she was indeed wounded by a spear – in fact it was a barbed fishing spear and it was still in her. She was sitting patiently in a chair by the charge nurse's office. It transpired that she had been fast asleep on her sleeping mat, when she was rudely woken, to say the least, by the impact of the spear. It had entered her cheek just below her left eye, and had exited about an inch and a half lower down. The spear had continued its flight however, and had gone into her again just behind the left collar bone. Somewhere down there it had embedded itself. The poor woman therefore had her face impaled and anchored by the spear to her body somewhere behind the collarbone.

Louis was out on tour so I was on my own in the station. You might have thought it would be a simple matter to withdraw the spear, but it was far from simple because there are several important structures behind the clavicle and first rib. I had no idea how long the end of the spear was, and therefore no idea how deeply it had gone into her. Neither did I know the pattern of the barbs on its end.

I took her into theatre. I wished Louis had not been on tour because anaesthetising her was not going to be easy – all we had was, as I said previously, the old rag and bottle anaesthetics, and in this case we couldn't put the mask over her face properly because of this great length of metal going through her cheek. I did my best to leave as much of the area round the nose and mouth for the anaesthetic mask as I could while still giving myself access to the wound.

Getting the spear away from the cheek was easy – all it needed was a small incision to free the shaft, and a couple of sutures to close up again. I took a deep breath before I started to explore the lower entry wound. This could be tricky, and could result, if I made a false move, in a severe if not fatal bleed. As carefully as I could, I separated the tissues, but the thing seemed as firmly stuck as ever. I gently probed to see if I could get some idea as to how far down it had gone – it seemed to go down forever. I had no idea how many twisted barbs there were, and I didn't dare go too deeply without being able to see where I was. I began to wonder if I was going to have to cut through the clavicle to make some space. Then suddenly, and to my immense relief, the shaft came out. Somehow I suppose I must have just twisted it in the right direction to free it. There was no bleeding, and I could only surmise that it had penetrated between the various anatomical layers without causing too much damage. We were all lucky that night. My patient healed up wonderfully well and soon went home. The next day the local police came to see me to ask me for a report on her injuries. They also asked for the spear. I had hoped to hang on to that as a memento of a fraught night's work. "Well," said the police superintendent, "you can have it after the case has been tried, but not until then. We are looking for the assailant, but he has gone." The attacker, it was thought, had fled to bush. So far as I know he never reappeared, so I never got 'my' spear. Perhaps it's as well. It was a fearsome thing, I must say.

Some of the most alarming things always seemed to happen at night, and often when Louis was on tour and I was on my own in station. About nine o'clock one evening, when I was just thinking how nice and quiet everything was and hoping it would remain so, the phone rang. This time it was not the hospital, but the Native Authority Health Representative in the town. "Doctor," he said, "I have had a message to say that two babies have been born joined together, and one has died. They are bringing them to you." My heart sank. The village from which they would be coming was 150 or more miles away. What on earth was I to do if the surviving babe was still alive on arrival? I had never even seen conjoined twins. There was no doubt but that I would be expected to do something when they came into Maiduguri. How I wished Louis were around, so that we could work together on this one.

I decided it wasn't worth trying to go to bed, and I waited up, trying to read or write letters to pass the time. I alerted the hospital, but really couldn't tell that what, if anything, would be done. I waited – and waited – and waited. No phone call. The hours passed. In the end I was so tired that I went on to my bed and must have crashed right out. When I woke it was morning. I dashed to the hospital – no ambulance had arrived in the night. Had it broken down on the road? What had happened? I rang the Health Representative. "Oh," he said casually, "One baby had died and the other baby died too, so they did not come." It seemed to be no big deal to him. I felt desperately sad for the mother, who would have endured what would probably have been a far from easy birth, only to see firstly that the babes were joined, and then to see both of them die, everything happening far from professional help.

Chapter 13

My first trip out of Maiduguri came along on 20th November 1957, about three months after I had arrived there. Not bush touring – that came later. This trip was to escort a patient by air from Maiduguri to Kano. My houseboys, Samuel and Amadu were full of importance in the knowledge that I was to be away, and they told me that they had organised themselves to do 'dayguard' on the house till I came back (as if they didn't watch it when I was at work anyway!). Samuel also asked me 'Will Madam ring the police and ask for a night guard?' I did, and he was happy. The expatriate Superintendent of Police (the Federal Nigerian Police) told me a lovely story afterwards about the police guard.

Returning to his own house when going off duty late one evening, he called round by my house to make sure that the constable was indeed there on duty. Yes, he was – sitting by my front door – but sound asleep.

The Superintendent spoke to him. He did not rouse.

The Superintendent removed his fez. He slept on.

The Superintendent removed his leather belt and his baton.

Still no response.

Finally, just as the Superintendent was about to drive off, with all the items of uniform that he had removed, the constable woke up.

'No thieves here Sir' he reported.

'No?' replied the Superintendent 'What about your uniform?'

And the constable suddenly discovered that he was missing several items.

I think the expected rocket was firmly delivered before the bits of uniform were returned.

This reminds me of another police story – again in Maiduguri, which I pass on as it was told to me by the same Superintendent. At the end of my road there was an empty house. There had been a spate of thefts on the GRA, and people reported hearing voices coming from this empty house at night. It was suspected that the thieves were using the house as a place to hide in during the evenings so that they were on the spot and ready to emerge late at night and do their breaking and entering. The Superintendent decided to do something about this, so one night his constables, in plain clothes, secretly and quietly surrounded this house and compound. They could indeed hear voices and see lights. Gradually they closed in, nearer and nearer, and finally they pounced...to find that the house was full of Native Authority police, sitting and gossiping instead of patrolling the station to ensure that all was well.

My trip to Kano was very pleasant. The patient survived his journey on the little local plane very well. Our pilot flew as low as he safely could so that any oxygen deprivation was kept to a minimum as there was no oxygen supply on the aircraft in case of emergency. Because we were so low, we had a very good view of the country below in spite of the haze of Harmattan which limited our visual range to about seven miles. Everything looked very dry, brown and dusty. From Maiduguri we flew first to Jos and then on to Kano where I handed my patient over to the local Medical Officer and was then free to follow my own devices.

There were only two aeroplanes a week into Maiduguri, so I had to wait until the next one went before I could get back. I was lucky therefore to have a few days in Kano. I had been booked into the Catering Rest House there, and having checked in, I contacted the nursing sister who had shared my cabin on the boat out from England. She was now in charge of the Nurses' Training School in Kano. I asked if we could meet and renew our acquaintance. Indeed we could, she said, and not only that – she cancelled my booking at the Rest House, insisting that I stay with her. More than that, she said that if I didn't mind running her to work in the morning and collecting her at the end of the day, I could have the use of her car to do shopping, exploring, whatever. What a difference this made to me, for I had inevitably been given long shopping lists by everyone I knew in Maiduguri, and I had been wondering how on earth I would cope with all the stuff I bought, or how I would manage to get to the canteens in the first place. When I did get the plane back to Maiduguri I had an enormous load to take back and had to pay huge freight charges as a result of the extra weight.

I found that Kano was big, busy and bustly, and I missed the relative peace and quiet of Maiduguri, not being a very 'towny' person myself. Actually, Maiduguri was not really quiet within the town, it had its various noises of course – voices, animal sounds, music played at night, and the sound of the open-air cinema when there was a film being shown. But Kano was so much more urban and in its way, sophisticated, whereas Maiduguri was far away from all that. I suppose having a big international airport helped to make Kano what it was. Surprisingly, our tiny airstrip in Maiduguri counted as an international airport officially, I was always told – possibly because you could, in the pilgrim season, fly to Mecca from there.

Although I soon tired of the urban-ness of Kano, I did enjoy the shops, which seemed to have an infinite variety of goods after the rather limited canteens that I had been buying from in Bornu, but shops are not the be-all and end-all of life. Kano, I felt, at least the parts of it that I saw and moved in, could have been almost any big city and I didn't feel that it typified Africa as I knew Africa, limited though my experience was as yet. It was more like Lagos – another big city with many shops, busy crammed roads and bustle. However, as I say, I really only saw part of Kano, and I didn't get into what was known as the *Sabon Gari* – the 'stranger's quarter', where the Southern Nigerians who worked in Kano all lived. I was to learn later that from time to time there was unrest involving the *Sabon Gari*, with discord between the Northerners and the Southerners. So far as I was concerned, everyone I met was very friendly, both in the town and back at Isobel's where I met several of her friends. We were invited out almost every evening while I was there and well entertained.

Although it was such a big place, Kano only had two hospitals. One was a large hospital in the middle of town for most of the local population, and the other was, like our nursing home in Maiduguri, for senior service personnel. Little did I think then that a couple of years later I would be a patient there myself, having my first child! However, at least Nassarawa Hospital was open all the time, unlike our nursing home in Maiduguri, which at that time was closed because of lack of staff. We only opened it up for an hour each day to hold a clinic. If any senior officer needed admitting it meant getting whoever it was through to Kano or even repatriating them. Later we were able to have it open all the time if needed, though for long periods we had no inpatients, and the staffing was never as good as we would have wished.

Kano airport was really quite big, and I am sure will be much bigger now. But when it was newly opened (and would have been very small), the Emir of Kano presented two camels to West African Air Lines, together with a ceremonial trumpeter. Camels and trumpeter would go out onto the tarmac to meet every incoming plane, and the arriving passengers would be greeted with a fanfare from the trumpet, and, I dare say, disdainful looks from the camels. The camels and presumably the trumpeter too were permanently housed at the airport. As the airport grew, the procession was stopped – there were just too many planes coming in for them all to be met. But the camels and trumpeters continued to live there and stationed themselves near to the tarmac so that they could be in full view of everybody, and I was delighted to have seen them myself, having heard so much about them.

My social activity continued in Maiduguri. Although I was working as hard as ever I did in the UK, I was having a social life like I'd never dreamed of in England. I think this was because in the absence of facilities like theatres, lectures, libraries and so on, we all did our best within our houses to entertain each other. I tried to play my part, though more than once when I was entertaining friends, I would be called down to the hospital. I would then ask the first arrivals to 'receive' for me and make everyone welcome. It was quite amusing to arrive later on at my own party and find that it was going with a swing!

I continued to go riding with a group of friends on days when I was not on call. Being on call meant that sometimes I couldn't ride for a week or two. When I finally got into the saddle again, I would be so stiff afterwards that I could hardly move the next day. But it was a great pastime and I always enjoyed it. I also went from time to time on long bush walks with another friend who went out to shoot game for the pot. He was very knowledgeable about the local wild life, so an outing with him was always fascinating.

Life was full, interesting and crammed with contrasts. I could spend all morning in the maelstrom of the hospital, dealing with the eternal clinics, going round the wards, operating or anaesthetising or dealing with administration in the office before dashing back to the wards or wherever. Then, occasionally I would forgo a siesta and would drive to the local market with its mass of people, noise and colour, heat, dust, and flies. One would wander among innumerable stalls, some selling lengths of materials, others displaying enamel plates and beakers, and yet others selling jewellery, bangles, ankle bracelets, beads, rings, all sorts. There would be the 'witch doctor's' stall, with little piles of strange looking substances, powders, crystals, bits of animal skins, you name it, it was there. Other stalls sold cosmetics – kohl for eye shadow (even the tiny girls had it put round their eyes), henna for dyeing hands and feet. This seemed to be very fashionable – you would see a woman with her hand and lower arm plunged into a long hollow gourd. She would keep it like that for several hours, for inside the gourd would be the henna mixture. When she took her arm out, her hand would have been dyed a bright orange colour.

You would hear the clicking of scissors in one area of the market – these would be from the barbers who opened and shut their scissors so that people would hear and know where to go to get their hair cut, or their heads shaved if they were Moslems. Further along, and usually positioned in a bit of shade were the tailors. You knew you were near them when you heard the unmistakeable sound of sewing machines stitching away. Singers (the manufacturers) must have done a huge trade in Nigeria! Many of the machines were old ones of the treadle variety, but others were operated by hand wheels. Every tailor was keen to pick up custom wherever and whenever he could. And at the edge of the market, in whatever shade they could find, the butchers set up their stalls. Although they all waved fly whisks around as much as they could, there was no stopping the dense clouds of flies around the raw meat. It looked very unappetising there, but our cooks still bought and cooked it. I suppose that roasted flies were pretty sterile, and we didn't seem to come to too much harm, though I was never much of a meat eater myself anyway. The butchering was like nothing we see here – one couldn't recognise cuts of meat as we know them in England, they were just chunks hacked off the animal more or less. There was plenty of fresh meat in Maiduguri because we were not in a tsetse area – that is why we had horses to ride and why there were the great herds of cattle moving about with their Fulani herdsmen. And there would be people selling other foods – fruit or vegetables, whatever was in season, or that had come up from farther south

Immediately outside the main market area one would see tethered animals, horses, donkeys, even the odd camel, all waiting patiently until their owners came for them. They would have been used to carry goods in for sale, or just to bring their riders in to buy goods. Some of the animals were lucky enough to be in patches of shade, but others seemed to have to stand all day in the hot sun. I felt very sorry for them. Smells there were in abundance – smells of animals, of people, of the rather rancid-odoured grease that some of the women used on their hair – smells of the pungent perfumes used lavishly by Kanuri men, especially important men. Everywhere one would smell dust, foodstuffs, even the heat. Maiduguri itself was actually an old walled town, with several gateways into it through the walls. To get to certain parts of the town one had to go through the main market area and out by a gate at the far side. I described another of my little forays into the town in a letter home:

'23.10.1957

I took myself a little trip round the native town the other afternoon instead of having siesta – all the people were going home from market & the streets were packed with people, donkeys, horses, cattle, strings of bulls etc. Down one side street I could hear music, so I turned the car down, & came across a little itinerant band – 3 drummers, all beating exciting rhythms, & a man playing a trumpet looking thing – but it was made of wood & had holes in it that you put your fingers on, & sounded like those little high pitched pipes playing weird tunes on about 3 notes only – you know the sort of thing I mean – you never hear that sort of music at home. I could have listened for a long time but as soon as they saw the car stop, they all came to play for me, & I could see myself having to distribute 'dash' all round – that means baksheesh or tips, so not having anything with me I had to drive on.
I also met a large mass of grass & leaves the size of a large haycock, with a little boy on top, travelling slowly along the road. Underneath it all, completely hidden but for its eyes & feet, was a donkey, doing all the work!!!! These poor patient donkeys.'

In contrast to the daytime colour, dust and noise, one could go for an evening walk, or just sit on the verandah at home for that matter, enjoying the last few seconds of the sunset with night coming up fast and the sky a lovely rich blue. Then, in minutes it would be pitch dark, and the sky like deep black velvet and the stars shining like no stars anywhere else. Sometimes there would be a full moon hanging there in the incredible stillness. Unforgettable. At such times you just did not notice the night-time whine of the mosquitoes – or their bites. There were other sorts of night-time sounds if you listened – the chirp of crickets, the croaking of frogs at certain times of the year. If you lived near to, or inside the African town as we did in Katsina later on, you might hear the sound of music late into the night, sometimes records, sometimes live African music, especially if an event was being celebrated. During Ramadan particularly, there would be a lot of noise from the town at night, for after sunset the people could eat and drink, and they made sure they enjoyed themselves during the hours of darkness, for at sunrise the fast had to be resumed. If you lived out towards bush, or even sometimes near to the town, there would be occasional animal cries as well.

I had heard people say that there were a lot of chameleons about, but I didn't actually see one for several months. Then, suddenly they seemed to be everywhere – perhaps there was a season for them. To my delight, one appeared on my verandah and took up residence amongst the coralita leaves. In the glow of the electric light from the lounge at night it took on the pale green – almost a creamy colour – of the leaves of the plant. It clung to the stems, motionless except for the swivelling of its eyes, and the sudden flash of its tongue when it shot out to catch a passing insect. My chameleon was really a very torpid animal and didn't seem to move much so long as it was left alone. If I went near it, it opened its mouth widely and hissed at me, coming out at the same time in alarming dark green spots (to frighten me, no doubt).

My houseboys were afraid of it, telling me that the breath of a chameleon would give you leprosy. I was sorry when one day it had gone. Had my boys dealt with it, or had it just decided to relocate? My boys were also afraid of lizards of which there was quite a variety in and around the house. There were the little pale geckos which ran up and down the lounge walls. There were bigger and rather brightly coloured ones in the garden and on the verandah. They seemed to know when I was having a post-siesta cup of tea and biscuits, and would run in through the open door to pick up any crumbs that I might drop. Needless to say I 'dropped' a lot, for I enjoyed seeing these little animals. They always ran outside again after their treat, scurrying away into the compound. What with chameleons, lizards and all the insects which lived in and around the house, life was never dull.

Insects were many and various. Some were intrusive, others almost self-effacing. Some seemed at times to be companionable and I quite missed them if they were not there.

The nightly high pitched whine of the mosquitoes will be familiar to anyone who has lived in the tropics. As soon as darkness fell, you'd hear the first of them and knew that it was time to put on the insect repellent. Before I sailed out, a friend of mine had said to me 'My dear, be sure to take plenty of pillow cases with you.' Pillow cases? Why, I wondered. 'Well,' she said, 'When I was in India, we used to put our feet into a pillow case in the evenings and pull it up over our knees. Kept the mosquitoes off our legs, you see.' In Nigeria I found that quite a lot of the expatriate women had made themselves long skirts to wear in the evenings (saved the pillow cases!) and almost everyone got themselves mosquito boots. I got some too, made for me by the local shoemaker in lovely soft leather. But actually I didn't wear them much because they were too hot. I relied on Dimp, which was the insect repellent of those days. It didn't help a lot, but it was effective for short periods.

There were lots of big flying jobs with hard wing cases which also appeared at night and banged themselves into windows and walls. I often thought they must give themselves dreadful headaches, for they never seemed to learn how not to hit hard surfaces in their flight. An insect that one had to be wary of was the cantharides fly. These were quite big, with green, almost iridescent wings – really rather beautiful. From time to time one settled on you. It was important to try to flick them off and not swat them on to yourself, for if you did that, then you finished up with a large and nasty cantharides burn from the juice that came from them. Often this was severe enough to make a huge and painful blister. Flies there were in abundance – not so many in my first house which was on the GRA, but in a later house on campus at the Training College which was on the edge of bush with cattle passing by not very far away there were no end of them. I remember using the Flit gun to spray the bedroom once, and counted fifty fly corpses afterwards. Five minutes later there seemed to be as many again already zooming round the room.

We had other insects too – strange praying mantises, beautiful butterflies, white ants which, if there was any woodwork in your house walls, managed to eat their way in through it, and then disappeared – by eating their way out again, I suspect. We also had wasps, hornets, and bees (all these with most fearsome stings, far worse than here in the UK). There were spiders, and scorpion-spiders (these were spiders which looked just like scorpions except that they had eight legs and no stinging tails). They were sometimes several inches long. We had sausage flies – these were like a huge sort of flying ant, and we only got them in the rainy season. Every so often in the evening there would be hundreds of them, flying into the lights and killing themselves as a

103

result. Our houseboys would hurry to shovel them up, for they fried and ate them as a delicacy.

And there were earwigs. These also appeared in the rainy season in their thousands. They would congregate often in the fuse boxes and fuse the electric circuits. They would block up taps by crowding into them. They got absolutely everywhere. When my children were babies, and before I changed their nappies, I had to shake out the pile of clean nappies and plastic pants to make sure they were not colonised by earwigs before I used them.

Once, after I was married, my husband had to fly to Kaduna for a conference at short notice. Kaduna was about 400 miles away. At the end of the conference, the powers that be, rather than expect him to wait several days before the scheduled return plane was due, laid on a small private plane to bring him back to Maiduguri. The pilot was a pleasant young American. They didn't arrive until late afternoon, and so, because there were no lights at the airport, the pilot stayed overnight with us. I hadn't known that we were to have a guest until they arrived, so while the two men were chatting, I hastily swept out the guest room, which was at the far end of the house from our bedrooms, and was self contained with its own door to outside and its en suite facilities. It was the rainy season at the time, so after I had made up the bed, I gave a quick spray round everywhere with the Flit gun, to clear out any insects.

In due course we all repaired to our various domains to bath and change before dinner. Later, while having our meal, I think I made some remark about how nice it was at the end of the day to freshen up and have a relaxed evening meal, and then I asked our guest 'Was everything all right for you?' Rather hesitantly, and with what one might call a bit of an old fashioned look, he replied that yes, everything had – er – been OK. I privately thought that if he had expected to find things as he would in uptown New York, he was expecting a lot. However, there were no more old fashioned looks and we spent a pleasant evening, sitting outside with our coffee and talking.

The next morning, our pilot was up bright and early, and all ready for his return flight to Kaduna. There had been some overnight rain and it was cool and fresh as we breakfasted, enjoying the after-rain smell that one only seems to come across in Africa. 'A purty day' commented the young man, 'Should be a nice flight'.

My husband drove him to the airport, while I, thinking to save the houseboys a little time, went through to the guest suite to strip the bed. I could not believe my eyes as I went in. All over the floor of the bedroom, bathroom and shower was a carpet of dead earwigs. The bath too was thickly lined with them as was the washbasin. Along the floor were the pilot's footprints, and in the bath I could see exactly how he had sat while washing, for there was a clear area in it. I was utterly astounded, and only then realised that the last thing I should have done was to have sprayed the rooms with insecticide, as it had brought out all the earwigs from the taps, water pipes, electric light switches and other nooks and crannies as they tried to escape the effects of the spray. I had never seen anything like it before and never have since. I forgave the young man his old fashioned looks, instead admiring him for his forbearance in not saying a single word about it.

I had discovered, incidentally, that many of the Africans I met didn't know a lot of the sort of natural history that I had learnt from childhood in England. If I asked the names of flowers, they couldn't tell me, even in Hausa – a flower was just a flower. Moreover, many could not, or did not, indicate colours by name, even in their own language. Of course there would be many who did know, but those with not much education really didn't seem to. I first realised this when one of the staff nurses at the hospital asked me to read the result of a urine test for sugar, because although he was not colour blind, he did not know what to call various colours. This astonished me, but there it was.

Chapter 14

I have said already how full the wards could be at the hospital, with extra 'beds' provided when necessary, which was almost always. When overfull, and so long as it was not the rainy season, we would first scrounge bedsteads from somewhere to put up out on the verandahs. When we had no more of those, we looked for spare mattresses, and nursed patients on the floor, and if the worst came to the worst, they had to be on sleeping mats – which for most of them would be what they used anyway so it was no hardship to them.

The children's ward was absolutely crammed full most of the time, with cots and beds all squashed up one against the other. There was no question of how many cubic feet per child – if they were ill enough to be in hospital, then into hospital they came and we just hoped for the best. It was sometimes like an obstacle course trying to get from one patient to another, especially when you remember that most of the mothers were there too! Children were admitted with all manner of ailments – ringworm, malaria, intestinal worms, anaemia, trauma, burns, scabies, malnutrition, you name it and it was there.

If there were any infectious diseases like measles, then we did have some old wards, very small ones which we used for 'isolation' wards. In fact these little buildings were condemned but had not been demolished. They had no running water or electricity like the rest of the hospital, and they were just behind the male outpatient clinic. Nevertheless, by dint of doing what we could in the way of barrier nursing, we managed to contain infections pretty well. I am sure that when the senior expatriate nursing staff or the medical officers were not on the spot, the barrier nursing was not exactly perfect, but still, we did our best. Each nurse donned a gown on top of his or her uniform, and washed hands in bowls full of disinfectant after tending to their patients. At least, that is what they did when we were around. At one time we had several cases of smallpox there. Daily I expected to see some spread, but Providence must have smiled on us, for the outbreak appeared to be contained. In another station I worked in, Katsina, we had a large concrete base at some distance from the main hospital. In the event of smallpox, the system was that grass matting walls and a roof would be erected and patients housed there. After any outbreak was over, the grass matting would all be burnt and the base well disinfected. Quite a good system. However, there was never any outbreak during my time there, luckily.

Further measures taken to try to prevent the spread of smallpox should it occur were the setting up of roadblocks on all roads out of Maiduguri. The roadblocks were manned by teams of vaccinators, who stopped vehicles and vaccinated the occupants forthwith. I am sure that this would not be foolproof however, for it would be no problem for foot travellers to make detours and bypass the road blocks by dodging round them through the bush. Also, the ever present system of 'dash' would mean that some people might pay the vaccinators not to do them or, alternatively, the vaccinators might demand payment for their services. I have earlier on described the problems we had over the vaccination of pilgrims who were making the annual Hadj to Mecca. Since that time, smallpox has been eradicated worldwide, so that somehow the message got through to even the remotest villages about the value and importance of vaccination. It was a thrill for me, years after I returned to the UK, to read the World Health Organisation reports of the successful campaign to stamp out smallpox. I have also elsewhere mentioned the fact that annually we anticipated an epidemic of meningitis. In order to try to control this, large quantities of sulphonamides were supplied to centres over the province, and in fact I don't recall any cases coming to us when I was in Maiduguri that first year.

The expatriate Health Sisters worked very hard indeed, for they spent a lot of time bush touring, setting up maternity and child welfare clinics in outlying places, advising on things like infant care, feeding and so on. The normal practice, I found, among the local mothers, was for babies to be breast fed until they were more than a year, sometimes eighteen months old. There was no gradual weaning as we know it, either you were breast fed, or you were old enough to eat grown up food. So really, the longer breast feeding could go on, the better. Young babies would not have coped with food that everyone else ate.

There was a great deal of tuberculosis to cope with in the general population. I had, in the first few years after I qualified and did my house jobs, worked a good deal with tuberculosis in sanatoria and chest clinics in different parts of the UK. Since my early days, when we saw really bad cases, we had seen the introduction of streptomycin and other medications for tuberculosis, and the badly advanced cases that I had seen at first simply disappeared and sanatoria were being closed down – in Britain. Now in Maiduguri I was seeing the sort of cases I thought I would never come across again. We treated people with all the right medication, and tried to keep them in special wards and therefore isolated from other patients. However, in spite of our trying to explain to them why they had to keep away from others, the lessons never seemed to sink in and one would find the TB patients wandering about the compound having a chat here and there with patients from other wards. Indeed, at one hospital where I worked, to my horror the women with TB did not have a ward of their own, but were nursed on the verandah surrounding the maternity unit. There was no other accommodation for them, and I worried about the new babies in the ward. We did not at that time have BCG vaccine available.

Neither did we have facilities for the treatments which were by that time discontinued in the UK – pneumothorax and the like. Moreover, from time to time we ran out of medication, and central stores did not send us what we had ordered, so that there were often long periods when we could not give our TB patients any medicines. At such times they would begin to drift home, and when we suggested that they should stay, explaining the nature of infection and the importance of all the other measures, their reply would be 'If there is no medicine, what is the point of staying here? We might as well go back to our homes.' Very few were persuaded to stay, even though many seemed to understand that unless they stopped being infective, they would simply pass the infection on at home.

In spite of the fact that there was an awareness that they were infectious, we knew that it was hard to persuade people to come to hospital with TB. They found that if their disease became known, people in their villages would shun them, so as you might imagine, they tried to keep it quiet. TB was a taboo subject, just as epilepsy was over here once – and on occasions still is, I think.

Another disease which we saw was leprosy. We didn't treat this at the hospital because the Mission doctor from Molai, which was a few miles out of Maiduguri, dealt with it in his local hospital. He came into Maiduguri each week to run a clinic in the town, and bad cases he admitted to his hospital. However, we did see cases from time to time in our clinics, but would refer them to him. The local people were apprehensive about leprosy and there was always somebody turning up in our clinics asking if we thought they had contracted it, and they would show us a patch of white skin, or say that they had an area of numbness that worried them. Sometimes they were correct in their fears, but at least they did come for help and treatment was possible. Many cases of leprosy were not infective and were allowed to remain at home and working.

My parents had asked me, amongst lots of other questions about my life overseas, what, if any, arrangements there were for religious services in Maiduguri. My mother, being a teacher, also asked about the education system. My father, who worked in Public Health, didn't ask me anything (probably very wisely, having read so many of my comments on local hygiene in the letters I sent home). I was able to tell them that apart from the local mosque there was an Anglican church, St John's, which was attended by an African congregation, though I was sure that any European who wished to attend would have been made very welcome. There was also a Roman

Catholic Church, which certainly was attended by several of the expatriates, one of whom was my colleague Louis Gonzalez. I would often see the priest as I was going home from the hospital at the end of the afternoon, strolling along the road by the church, breviary in hand, enjoying the last of the daylight and the slightly cooler air as the sun at last went down.

The small courthouse on the GRA was used on Sundays as a church by many of the expatriate officers. One of the Molai Mission staff would come in on Sunday evenings to conduct our service. If there was anybody clerical at the Mission, he would take it, but otherwise the medical officer would officiate, or the manager of the Mission bookshop which was in Maiduguri, near the canteens. Various members of the congregation would read the lessons, and a list of those willing to take part in this was always organised in advance. Like many others, I took my turn with the readings. On Sunday mornings a small Sunday School would also be held there which was taken during my time by several members of the expatriate staff from the Government Girls' School. I thought it was nice for expatriate children to be brought together each week in that slightly formal setting, for there were no schools for them in the station, other than (and only occasionally if any wife was interested enough to run one) a tiny nursery group. Children of school age either went to boarding school in the UK or, if they attended primary school there, then their mothers would have to go back to the UK with them and those families would only be together during the odd holiday times for a few weeks. I learnt some time after we came home on retirement that permission had been withdrawn for the courthouse to be used as a church. This was after Nigeria had become fully independent, and also after the first uprising that preceded the Biafran war.

Finally there were the pagan tribes. They mostly lived out in bush areas some considerable distance from Maiduguri. I am not qualified to discuss their beliefs, for I knew and still know, so little about them. I was always told that they would be hostile to Europeans, as most lived in 'unsettled' areas. I doubted that things were as bad as that really – after all, the Health Sisters went into some remote areas. The pagans lived very differently from the Hausa and Kanuri people, hunting and defending themselves with bows and arrows, and generally wearing nothing but a bunch of leaves fore and aft, in contrast to the Kanuris and Hausas, who wore quite elaborate and often colourful dress. However, the pagans whom I did meet seemed a friendly lot and it would have been nice to have learned more about them.

The educational arrangements were a mixture of institutions. There were primary schools, run by the Native Authority. Some of these were in the town, while others were situated in outlying villages all over the place. There was a local Native Authority Education Officer who kept an eye on these schools, and he in turn worked with the Government Provincial Education Officer (PEO), who was a sort of director of education, and who had overall responsibility for the running of schools in his Province. This meant that the PEO had an office in the provincial headquarters (in our case, Maiduguri), and dealt with all the administration, as well as regularly inspecting the local schools. Outlying schools over the rest of the province also had to be regularly checked by the PEO, who therefore had a heavy and demanding touring programme to cope with in the dry season. It was a tough job really, for there was only one PEO to deal with everything, whereas for us at the hospital it was a lot easier, because when one of us was out of station, the other could keep all the administration and other hospital work going as usual.

The other (more senior) educational establishments were all boarding schools or colleges and were run directly by Government. The PEO had to liaise with the Principals of these institutions too. There was a Women's Teacher Training College (known as the WTC); the Provincial Girls' School (known as the PGS); and the Middle School, which became the Provincial Boys' Secondary School while I was there, and which was moved out of its original buildings into a fine newly built customised campus on the Airport Road. There was the Government Craft School, also built during my time in Maiduguri, and also on the Airport Road. And finally there was the Men's Teacher Training College (The Bornu Training College), which also occupied a fine campus next door to the Boys' Secondary School. This only began in 1960, but more of its story later on.

These boarding establishments were all (when I first went out there) headed by expatriate officers, although the staff complement would be made up of both indigenous and expatriate teachers and lecturers. After Independence, the policy was to replace expatriates with African staff, and indeed, when we left Nigeria for good, my husband, who was the first Principal of the Bornu Training College, was replaced by a Nigerian Principal. I will write more about the schools system later on in this account, however, as I became closely involved with it in the fullness of time when I was asked to organise a school and college medical service. For the time being I simply saw scholars and students at the hospital in my normal clinics.

I think I should also mention the Koranic schools, though these were not connected in any way with the Native Authority or the Government. They were run by 'Mallams' who taught the children the Koran. The schools that I saw mostly were groups of children sitting under trees by the roadside as I drove to and from the hospital. They would sit in a circle with their teacher, and each held a board on which was written the Koranic passage for that day. They would rock back and forth as they chanted the text, until, presumably, they could remember it all. I supposed that they had a fresh text each day

110

and thus eventually learned the whole lot. With the car windows always open, I could hear the children's chant as I passed them. When I was going home in the early afternoon, and the heat was at its height, they would all be lying down in what shade they could find, sleeping. Later in the day, when it got cooler, I was told that the children then had to set to and prepare their meals, including food for their teacher. I never knew where they slept at night – did they go home to their families, or did they live with their teacher? What happened to them when they grew up? Did they in turn run their own little Koranic schools, or did they look for other work? I didn't find out then and I don't suppose I shall ever know now.

Chapter 15

Some people I had become friendly with in Maiduguri kept two rather nice dogs – a cross between spaniels and red setters, I think they were. The bitch was about to have pups, and I was promised one of these. He duly arrived at my house several weeks later and soon endeared himself not only to me but also to my houseboys, who spoilt him rotten. This was surprising, for with rabies being endemic in the country, and lots of bush dogs all over the place (everyone called them pye-dogs), the locals didn't as a general rule take to canines and rather treated them with suspicion and avoidance.

We – or I – had a bit of a problem at first with the task of house training my puppy. Not wanting him to wander away and get lost before he knew where he belonged, he had to be confined to the house to start with. So I organised a litter tray inside, and told the boys that 'if the little dog makes a mess on the floor, show it what it has done and put it in the tray' (to give the pup the message of where it should go for these purposes). However, the boys got completely the wrong end of the stick. Certainly they told me that they had 'shown the little dog what it had done' – but 'putting it in the tray' meant something quite different to them. When I got home, I found little puddles all over the floor, and little parcels with unmentionable contents carefully wrapped up and put tidily in the litter tray! It took quite some time before my pup knew to go outside at appropriate times.

Although things were still very hot as compared with what they would be in Britain, the fact that we were now in Harmattan meant that we could kid ourselves that we were having 'winter', all seasonable for Christmas. The temperature would drop at night from around 90 degrees F to about 75 degrees F, and I for one felt really cold, needing to have a blanket on my bed, and wearing a woolly cardigan first thing in the morning. If I went out for dinner anywhere in the evenings, I was able to wear a long sleeved dress and a petticoat and nylon stockings – and I would also take a woollen stole with me in which to wrap myself up as the evening wore on. What a difference. The dust laden wind at this time cut down visibility, and gave the effect of a thick mist. In the house, even if you kept windows and doors shut, the dust seeped in everywhere. No amount of dusting or sweeping inside seemed to make any difference and everything looked awful all the time. Wooden ornaments had to be wrapped up and put away so as to prevent them (hopefully) from cracking with the dryness. Many people found that their skin even peeled out of sheer dryness, even the Africans. One's hair got very dry as well, and full of dust, yet to wash it took any natural grease out and made it drier still. I started to put oil on mine after washing it – I'd never had to do that before – in the hopes that it would counteract the dryness, though it never did.

The Koranic students still sat under the trees, but now they were all wrapped up in blankets, and I noticed that they stayed awake for much more of the day instead of sleeping beneath the neem trees in the afternoons.

I have earlier mentioned the itinerant traders who, like travelling pedlars of times gone by in England, would appear from nowhere to sit on your doorstep, opening their packs and displaying their wares in the hopes that you would spend a lot of money. The name of the game was haggling over prices. I'd never done this before and it seemed strange to me. However I soon got the idea that it was really rather fun for all concerned, and certainly it was expected of you. The trader always asked far more than he expected, and you would counter by offering far less than you would actually pay in the end, but in fact this preliminary skirmish told you both the approximate end point of the negotiation. One soon learned how to pitch one's first offer, and the end result I feel sure always worked satisfactorily for both parties. The rest was, as I said, really a bit of a game. The traders came round regularly and in the end one almost regarded some of the regulars as friends. One in particular, who spoke quite good English was an interesting man and a cut above the others, I always thought. He was always happy to sit on the doorstep with me and discuss all sorts of world affairs, or local politics, or indeed any subject one cared to introduce, and he had useful views to offer as well. Somehow I felt that it was almost immaterial to him whether he actually sold me anything or not, though probably he always hoped for a sale. But I did have some of my better buys from him.

One day when he came, he told me that his brother ('same mother same father' he said, as opposed to 'brother' meaning somebody from the same village) was a patient at the hospital and in my care. Could he, he asked politely, give me some money (and he offered me £5) to make sure that his brother had the best treatment? I told him that I always did my best for any patient under my care and that he did not need to pay me any extra. In any case, I said, I was paid by Government to do my job. He could be assured that I was already doing everything I could for his brother as well as for anyone else for whom I was responsible. I thanked him for his offer, but declined it. 'Very well then' was all he said, but I was secretly amused to note that on a subsequent visit to my house he charged me less for the items I bought than he had ever done before. I guess he felt that he had satisfied his own honour in that way.

Out of the traders' packs, I had already managed to find Christmas gifts for my family back in the UK. From the same traders I bought things for myself too – a head harness for a horse, with leather fringes that would shake and keep flies out of the horse's eyes, a knife, a spear head, skin mats for my house. I also bought several 'Timbuktu' blankets which I occasionally used as floor coverings. These were rough hand-woven woollen blankets made by stitching together long woven strips with earth-coloured designs in the weave.

Shortly before Christmas, I invited the senior members of the hospital African staff – the equivalents of ward sisters, theatre staff and staff nurses, to my house one afternoon for tea and mince pies and the nearest I could get to Christmas cake. I didn't know if anyone else did this kind of thing, but I felt that if so, then I wasn't letting the good name of the expatriate doctors down; and if not, then it might be something new for our nurses to come across. It seemed to me that it was very new to them. They were a mixture of Southerners, who would be mostly Christian, either Catholic or Anglican, and Northerners who to a man (and woman) would be Moslem. Along they came, all together in one big group. I had amassed all the chairs in my house in the lounge, and almost everyone got a seat. Those without sat on the floor.

Dressed in their best outfits, caftans and *rigas*, with the women in colourful head dresses, except for the Kanuri women whose head adornments were their unique hair styles, they sat in almost total silence, nobody knowing what to say. Conversation was not easy, but I tried my best and we did get some sort of talk going, but it was stilted.

Everyone accepted a cup of tea and drank it, but although I saw not one person eat, every last mince pie and piece of cake disappeared. I think they must all have put the eats in their pockets to take home and show to their families. After what I suppose was considered to be a 'decent interval', the senior charge nurse stood up and thanked me on behalf of them all, and they trooped off back down to town, again all in a group together. I was glad they had felt able to come, although there never being any feedback, I never knew what they had thought of it all. It was the strangest Christmas party I had ever held!

About ten days before Christmas, Louis went out on his first bush tour, leaving me in charge of the hospital, which meant that in addition to coping with all his clinical work as well as my own, I also had to spend time in the office on the administration. I decided to go into the office first thing and clear the desk, after which the next couple of hours was spent on clinical duties before I returned to the office for another quarter of an hour to deal with all the things which had accumulated for me since I'd been there earlier. I would make a final office visit just before going home, when (hopefully) everything else was finished, so that (again hopefully) the desk would have been cleared altogether for that day leaving nothing hanging over for the morrow. It didn't always work out like that of course, for so often I was held up with either ward or outpatient work, and by the time I got back to the desk, the clerks would have gone home and locked up.

In the intervening time I seemed to be dashing round everywhere. If the wards were not busy (or even when they were), I would find that there were still outpatients waiting to be seen – people that the nursing staff could not themselves deal with. And there would always be stuff for theatre. Louis and I never arranged any cold surgery if one of us was out on tour because planned cases could sometimes be quite big operations for which it was better to have two doctors so that one of us could give the anaesthetics. But there was always surgical work coming in – small emergencies, sometimes big ones, which had to be dealt with whether there were two doctors available or not. Some things could not wait.

One of the first things I had to cope with in this way was an emergency Caesarean Section. Although I had anaesthetised and assisted at many such cases back in the UK, I had never actually done one myself. However, there was nothing else to be done but to get on with it now. I was secretly very pleased when the African nurse who anaesthetised for me told me how quickly I had done it. He had no idea it was the first time for me and his jaw dropped when I told him. The patient recovered normally I am happy to say, so my 'first' had been a success.

Not long before Christmas, the Maiduguri Post Office ran out of stamps. This was a blow, as I for one was all ready to send off my Christmas cards, each of which normally only needed a single penny stamp. The Post Office clerk decided that as there were no proper stamps left, he would cut out the fourpenny ones which were printed on airmail letters, for which he then charged the full fourpenny price. I wondered about the legality of using cut-out stamps in this way, but as all my cards seemed to arrive safely, it seemed that the authorities concerned had turned a blind eye to that practice.

It could only happen in Africa! Different, anyway.

On Christmas Day itself, Matron, Louis and I went round all the wards at the hospital giving a gift to every patient. There was a packet of sugar, a bar of soap and some sweets for each of the men, and a blouse and necklace for each of the women. Non-Moslem men also had a few cigarettes given to them. The children's ward was the best, so we saved that till last. Each child was given sugar, sweets, a toy and either a comic or a small scrap-book, a balloon, and a penny. Every child's pack of gifts came off the Christmas tree which had been put up in the ward. The children were so excited and jumped about and chattered twenty to the dozen. They had all learnt to say 'Merry Christmas', but had been defeated by 'Father Christmas', giving him instead the title of 'Mallam Christmas'. 'Mallam' is a courtesy title, inferring education and learning. A schoolmaster would be a Mallam.

I wrote about Christmas Day to my parents, telling them particularly of 'our little bush boy' (from pagan country, he was,) who, until he came to the hospital, had never seen a white person. At first he was terrified of us all, but soon lost his fear and was now so much at ease that he was imitating our English speech. He never got the words right, but managed the intonation so well that you could almost believe he was speaking English. The only word he could reproduce properly - and this he did very clearly - was what the nursing sisters affectionately called him - 'cheekyface'. I wrote to my parents:

'26 December 1957

...I can see a day when a rather proper and very British District Officer will be going through some outlying bush country one day, and will be greeted as 'cheekyface' by a little pagan wearing his bunch of leaves fore and aft, and will he [The District Officer] get a shock!'

The little boy had come in to us because following an injury some weeks previously, his arm became gangrenous and most of it dropped off, leaving a nasty unhealed stump, part of which I amputated a couple of days after Christmas, and tidied the rest up for him. The dropping off of most of his arm probably saved his life in fact, as if the gangrene had spread it would have killed him. This sort of thing happened quite often.

I was starting to think about things I would like to buy for myself, but for which I would have to start saving. The colour and movement all around me made me wish I had a cine-camera - you could not buy colour films for ordinary cameras yet - or if you could, you certainly could not in Maiduguri. But for cine-cameras, yes, colour film was obtainable, and the colour was good too. I also began to long for a record player and some records so that I could have music to listen to. Up till then, the only way in which record players - electric ones that is, could be played in stations where there was no electricity (and there were many of these) was by hitching them to one's car battery. In such places, therefore, if one decided to have some music, one had to settle probably for a 'dead' car battery which would need a good deal of help from friends before it could be brought to life again. In Maiduguri we did have an electricity supply so that record players could be plugged in to a socket, so long as the power was not cut off. It wasn't until I had been out for some months that we saw the first record player run off small dry batteries - and that was like magic to everyone. Louis, who was a grand opera addict, was thrilled when one of our nursing sisters came back off leave with a small player powered by dry batteries. He promptly commandeered it to take out on tour with him, saying that he looked forward to having the music sung at full volume out in bush. I wrote to my family that such magical things existed, adding that "They are worked with, of all things, five small torch batteries, and you get about 100 hours on that!"

Real up to date stuff, that was. I also very much wanted a typewriter because my mother constantly complained that she could not read my writing and that Dad had to interpret my letters for her. But all these things cost money.

A few weeks later on it was my birthday and I planned to host a drinks party for all the people who had entertained me. I was amazed at the length of the list, and had to send my boys all over the station to borrow glasses for the event, as I only had about half a dozen of my own. We were all accustomed to seeing our wine glasses and so on appearing at different parties! After that, I thought things would settle down into a nice quiet routine.

The first 'nice quiet routine' event was that, early in January 1958, Samuel, my cook-steward, gleefully announced to me one morning that he would be leaving within a couple of days as his previous employer was returning from leave and wanted him back. It was the first time I had known that Samuel was on a retainer for somebody else and not to be permanently in my employ. This was a blow, for we, the boys and I, had all settled together well. For the time being, therefore, I was thankful for my little camping petrol stove and on it I cooked my evening meals. Amadu got going like a little trooper and coped with my breakfasts and lunches (fruit salads and occasionally a bit of toast), and he worked hard in the house too and kept it looking really nice. I was very lucky in the end, because my expatriate next-door neighbour was returning to his own country, and his cook therefore was going to be out of a job. My neighbour recommended him to me, saying that he was a superb cook. And that is how Ali Katsina came to me. He was indeed superb – like an African Jeeves, quiet, unobtrusive, very responsible and reliable, honest, hard working – and a marvellous cook. He acted for me as cook-steward, and ran the house like a dream. He was married with a sweet little wife, Asumi, and two little boys, Mohammed and Garba, who would wave shyly and giggle at me if they saw me in the compound. When I married later on, and my husband and I had to sort out our respective house staff, we asked Ali if he would stay as cook and head boy and we were delighted when he agreed. He remained with us right until we left Nigeria on retirement and we felt that he was really part of the family in the end.

The next 'quiet routine' event was the visit of the Governor of Northern Nigeria, Sir Gawain Bell, and his wife in early January 1958. They were making a great tour all round the region, which Sir Gawain probably did every so often. He was an important personage, the direct representative of the Queen, just as the Resident was her representative in Maiduguri, so this was to be a big occasion. It was exciting therefore to be invited to a

117

reception and cocktail party at the Residency hosted by Sir Gawain. The party was held out on the lawn (the Residency being one of the few places in Maiduguri which actually had a lawn with real grass). As it was Harmattan and the evenings were cool, a brazier had been lit in the middle of the lawn and gradually everyone gravitated to it for warmth. The only problem was that there was just the one brazier and about a hundred and fifty of us! It was fun having one's name announced as one arrived, and then filing past Sir Gawain and Lady Bell who shook our hands and welcomed us. Occasions like this had not been part of my life in England. Earlier in the day they had visited the hospital where Louis and I had been formally introduced to them. Actually we were very glad that the visit didn't last too long, as on formal occasions like that, men were expected to dress in suits and ties, and women had to wear stockings, hats and gloves and in that heat it was torture! Poor Lady Bell must have been very uncomfortable as she would have to wear formal clothes a great deal of the time. We at least could rip off our stockings (together with the accompanying suspender belts - no tights in those days) and gloves as soon as she had gone. You only had to walk a few yards on the gritty sand to have nylon or silk stockings torn to shreds anyway, and they were not items of wear that you could buy in Maiduguri. I for one hoped that there would not be too many more formal occasions before I went on leave, as I'd only brought one or two pairs of stockings to Africa with me.

On the day the Governor arrived, district heads and chiefs from all over Bornu went to the airport to meet and greet him. They had to pass the hospital on their way out of town. The procession took roughly an hour to pass. It was the most colourful thing I'd ever seen in my life! I was working in the male outpatient clinic, and saw it all through the clinic window which was not more than ten yards away from the road. How I wished I'd had a camera with me.

Each chief was mounted, and was preceded by about thirty men walking abreast, all dressed in brilliant colours. These men held horsehair flywhisks which they twirled in set patterns that fitted into the rhythm of accompanying music. In turn each line of men was preceded by either a jester who jumped and danced about, or by a single horseman. The jesters and riders were dressed to represent something to do with their particular districts - for example, one man wore a head-dress like the head of a crown bird.

The chiefs themselves were dressed in magnificent robes and turbans of all colours, some with glistening gold turbans. They held shining swords and spears that glinted in the sun as they were waved and shaken in salute. Their horses were caparisoned in wonderful trappings, some of which were embroidered and decorated most elaborately, with even the backs of the horses covered right down to the ground as if they had trains behind them.

118

Made me think of pictures of medieval knights. The animals had brilliant head harnesses with bright tassels on them that looked like so many rainbows when the animals tossed their heads. Some also had beautifully chased silver collars on, and silver decorations on other parts of their harness.

A few horses had what looked like trousers, on either front or back legs. One of them had scarlet 'trousers' on all four legs, and I was told that it was the only one allowed to be dressed in that way, by virtue of its owner's office – he was something important in the Ministry of Defence.

Several of the chiefs wore overgarments of chain mail – said to have come from the Crusades. Could they really have survived for so long? I was willing to believe everything I was told. Behind each chief came the musicians, blowing long silvery trumpets that only produced two or three notes, but the combination of these notes was captivating and haunting.

Finally, bringing up the rear of each chief's retinue came the remainder of his men, all similarly mounted and caparisoned, and their parades stretched behind for a considerable distance before the next chief's display began. District after District came by in this manner. It was fairytale stuff – Arabian Nights come to life.

And on all sides this wonderful procession was accompanied by people from the town, mounted, on bicycles, on foot, anyway they could get, running alongside trying to keep up.

And here I must report a slice of good luck that had come my way not long before the Governor's visit. I mentioned earlier that my next door neighbour was returning to his own country, and that I had taken on Ali, his cook. My neighbour had also said to me (he had known that I was saving up for a cine-camera) – "I have both a cine-camera and a projector. I don't want to take them back home – would you like to buy them second hand from me? They are both in good condition." Would I like them? Indeed I would. In two or three minutes, and at a ridiculously small cost, I was their proud owner, and when I realised that there would be a durbar, I dashed to Norchem (the only chemist's shop in Maiduguri) and bought their last two 8mm cine-films, on which I was able to record some of the display.

Louis, bless his great heart, had told me, "Off you go, girl – I'll look on for the hospital. I've seen durbars before – this will be your first one. Don't miss it."

The Shehu, by then about 85 years old and with failing eyesight, the Waziri and other Native Authority officials, the Governor and Lady Bell, the Resident and Mrs Letchworth, all sat immediately in front of the entrance to the palace on a little platform. Stretching away in front of them was a huge empty area, the Dandal Way – which seemed to me to be as big as Horse Guards Parade in London. The same processions we had seen going to greet the Governor on his arrival had all massed out of sight at the far end of the Dandal Way, and now, district by district, they came into sight and processed down towards the palace, first those on foot, all abreast, followed by similar lines of horsemen who were led by their District chiefs. Just in front of the dais they stopped and saluted by waving their swords and spears, flywhisks and anything else they had to wave, before riding away to the side and out of sight.

Then, after every District had gone by, came the grand finale. From the far end of the Dandal Way, there suddenly burst a group of galloping horseman, going full gallop and then some. Nearer and nearer they came, faster and faster, or so it seemed, right up to within a yard or two of the Shehu and his party. At that point, they suddenly reined in their horses, some of which almost sat down on their hind legs with the speed of the sudden halt. Very dramatic. One always felt that they wouldn't be able to stop in time and that the VIP party would be mown down and cut to bits by flying hooves. But the riders always stopped in time and nobody was ever hurt. It was terrific. No Hollywood film could beat it. The governor, for whom the whole thing had been laid on, stood to greet all the riders and the people who had come, some from very far away – Bornu was a huge province – and he in turn saluted them and thanked them all before being driven back to the Residency, accompanied by Native Authority Police outriders (horseback again) with their bright fezzes, and pennants flying from poles stuck in the stirrups. A brave sight it all was.

And then the crowds drifted gradually away, leaving the Dandal Way empty as before, with just one or two groups of dancing women left to entertain anyone who wanted to watch. I was always told that the dancers were the local ladies of the night, but all I can say is they put on a good show in the daytime, too, with their wonderful garments and (if they were Kanuri) their strange hair styles.

More than forty years later I was to see in a magazine a small reproduction of a picture painted by Peter Kuhfeld, an artist who had been invited to accompany the Prince and Princess of Wales on a formal visit to Nigeria. The picture, to my great pleasure, was of a durbar in Maiduguri. As I looked at it, I was in my mind transported back there, scuffing my feet on the gritty sand, and feeling the sun beat down mercilessly on us all during the hottest part of the day. I could once again hear the sounds – the strange music, the fanfares, the jingling of the horses' accoutrements, the rush of the galloping hooves and the sounds of the crowds as they shouted their salutes. I could smell the smell of the dust again, and of the pungent scent which the Kanuri men used. And I could hear once more the soft whirr of my little cine-camera as I tried to capture it all on film.

120

Louis now prepared to go out on tour. We used the last week before he went as well as we could, clearing the wards of all planned surgery, dealing with things like hernias, hysterectomies, removal of fibroids, amputations of limbs affected by tropical ulcers, as well as anything in the way of minor surgery that was lying about waiting to be done. One never knew what would present itself next, so it was vital to keep up with things and keep the decks cleared for action. Louis in his usual generous way, insisted on taking all calls, day or night, in that last week so that I could have a good rest before I was left to carry the hospital on my own until his return. So I had a lovely week, able to accept invitations out, go riding, get all my bulk shopping done and generally relax.

One of the parties to which I was invited that week was held by a French couple. The husband was in charge of the canteen CFAO (Compagnie Française de l'Afrique Occidentale), where, incidentally I had spotted a typewriter for sale – an Olivetti Portable model, and had snapped it up. I still have it, though I can no longer get ribbons for it and I doubt that even if I could, it would function now after so many years. The invitation came in the form of a poem, written in French. I managed to translate it with the help of a tiny French/English dictionary I had. At the bottom of the card was written 'RSVP (*Français* of course)'. I determined to reply in French if I could, and then thought 'I wonder if I could manage a bit of doggerel in French?' it seemed fun to try anyway, so with remnants of my school French, last studied twenty years before, I had a go. On the night of the party, we found that all our replies had been pinned up on the wall, and mine was the only one in rhyme, which caused more than a little amusement. Thereafter, whenever I met my host anywhere, he would command me, sotto voce, "*Parle Français!*"

My orthopaedic efforts progressed. The Mammy wagon accidents continued to flow in. One particular patient from such an accident came in with both femurs fractured and also both lower legs. He was really smashed up. One leg was practically hanging by a thread and the other had open fractures. We took him straight into theatre where I thought at first I was going to have to amputate. However, after a bit of manipulation under anaesthesia I managed to get the bone ends together and fixed them by screwing metal plates (all we had) across the fractured ends, and I also managed to sort out the soft tissue trauma. I noted in my letter home that the resulting position was not exactly perfect and that his leg in future would not be totally straight, but 'at least,' I wrote 'it's still on him and not in the incinerator.' Back on the ward I managed to fix him up with various kinds of traction to get both legs into pretty fair positions, so that if he healed up well, he would be able to walk again, which he eventually did. The nursing staff had been very interested

121

in all the procedure, as they had never seen any of the apparatus used that I had dug out of the theatre cupboards. I was really thrilled myself, and eternally grateful to the orthopaedic surgeon, Reggie Tatham, with whom I had worked at Beverley, and who had taught me so much by example. From being totally 'physician minded' I had come to enjoy surgery quite a lot and in particular orthopaedics.

My puppy had grown into a grand little dog, a good companion, full of fun, and quite a good 'look-out' dog for me as well. He was joined by the dog from next door, which, when my neighbour left, simply walked across the compounds and elected to live at my house. This suited everyone because the new man next door did not like dogs, and my pup was already friends with our new arrival, whom I called Sandy. My pup, Cash, loved to go in the car, and if ever he thought I was going out, he would go and stand hopefully by the passenger door, wagging his tail and waiting to get in. Sandy was much more of a bush dog, and was terrified of motors, refusing at all times to be transported by car. They were both due for their rabies vaccinations now. No prizes for guessing which of them came happily with me to the Veterinary Department and which had to be visited at home by the vet for their jabs. It was also starting to be the tick season, which meant that each day I had to search them and then de-tick them as appropriate. Despite all the vigilance, Cash got tick fever twice over the years and was extremely ill both times. The vet saved him each time, and I was surprised at the speed of his recovery once he had had his antibiotics. Why did I call him 'Cash'? Well, before I set sail for Nigeria, a friend of mine said to me "I bet you'll get married out there."

"I jolly well bet I won't – I shall have far too much to do otherwise," was my response, so we had a £1 bet on it. And so my little dog was named 'Cash' – to remind me not to lose that bet.

A few weeks later I also got my horse 'Market Boy'. He had been a racehorse initially, but was deemed to be too slow, so I had the use of him for hacking. He was a very pretty animal with kind eyes, tending to take off at times if he got excited, but on the whole, at first, he was very biddable. However, (and I suspect the horse boy had been feeding him too many oats) he started to be very frisky and far too strong for me, and sadly I had to let him go. Doctors were not all that plentiful on the ground for one to risk being injured in a riding accident. In any case, I was really far too busy at the hospital to be able to ride regularly, so perhaps it was all for the best. I think in the end he was taken once more into racing.

Although I bought dry goods of all sorts and drinks from the local canteens, and my cook bought things like meat, flour, fruit and vegetables (if there were any), in the local market, I was able to buy eggs and chickens from the hospital food contractor. Eggs were tiny, almost as small as bantam eggs, and we would use four or five to make one omelette. I suppose therefore that I was a good source of revenue to the contractor, as I seemed to live on omelettes, not being all that fond of meat. One day however, I had ordered a chicken from him – probably because I was having people in for dinner that evening. The contractor said that he would leave it at the office for me to collect when I went home. On finally finishing my work therefore, I returned to the office to collect my fowl. There was nothing in my office anywhere, and in fact everybody but Mr Sofosu, the chief clerk, had already gone home, and he was just on the point of locking up for the day.

"Have you seen the contractor?" I asked, "I ordered a chicken and he said he'd leave it here for me." Mr Sofosu looked doubtful. No, he hadn't seen the contractor at all. Then he brightened up a bit – "But there was a chicken walking about outside earlier," he told me. Walking about? Couldn't be mine, I thought, for mine would be killed, trussed and ready for the oven, wouldn't it? We looked outside. Sure enough, there was a rather bedraggled chicken pecking disconsolately in the sand outside the office. I noticed that its legs were hobbled, loosely tied together with some string. "Yes, that's the one," said Mr Sofosu, picking it up and putting it in the back of my car, where it flapped and clucked all the way home. Being so new to the country, I had not until then taken on board the fact that one bought chickens alive, for once killed, the heat soon affected them so that they were not fit to eat. The poor things had to be freshly killed for the pot, which meant that one's cook did the honours, not the contractor who sold them.

Writing this reminded me of a time several years later, when it was Christmas. My cook Ali came to tell me that one of the college food contractors had left us a gift of three turkeys. "One woman, two man," said Ali, and there they were, wandering about in the compound, the 'woman' looking, I thought, a bit fed up with her two 'men'. We had a bumper Christmas that year for food!

Chapter 16

At the beginning of March 1958, the time came for me to start my bush touring. Louis had planned two trips out for me, one down to Biu, near the foothills of the Northern Cameroons and about 180 miles out of station. The second foray would be in a northerly direction almost up to the border of the Sahara, to a place called Nguru.

To my regret he did not let me do a third trip up to the northeast of Bornu, as that area was said to be unsettled as yet and not safe for a woman to go on her own. If I were a man, I was told, and could use a revolver, I would be allowed there. I was disappointed, but it couldn't be helped. I never heard of anyone getting into problems with these unsettled areas, but orders were orders and had to be obeyed.

A week beforehand Ali, who would accompany me and who would attend to my creature comforts while I was away as well as acting as interpreter on the journeys, started to put together all the things we would need – tinned food, crockery and cutlery, my camp bed, mosquito poles and net, camp stove and a folding canvas bath which I borrowed from my opposite neighbour the vet, a Tilley lamp which I borrowed from Louis, and (but not until the moment when we departed) the water filter from my kitchen. Young Amadu, who was to be left in charge of the house and dogs, and who took these duties and responsibilities very seriously, spent the week rehearsing all the extra things that he would need to do while he was my temporary major-domo. I wrote in my weekly letter to my parents:

'Maiduguri
26.2.1958

...Amadu is busy this week taking charge of the dogs' food, so that I can see if he knows how to look after them properly, and Louis is going to pop in from time to time, and also send his boy round to give a guiding hand to Amadu who after all is only a young boy and I should think it will be the first time he has been left 'in charge', for what it is worth, all he will have to do really is to feed the dogs and tell any visitors that I am on tour. He may do a bit in the house, but I think most likely he will stay in his little house [the boys' quarters were on the compound] and talk to his friends! Ali would be different, and would probably spring clean while I was out of the way, as he never leaves himself idle,

124

I notice he always finds something to do, unlike a lot of boys.'

I was told that I might just see some animals on the road – chiefly baboons, but perhaps leopard or even the odd lion. However the latter, it seemed, didn't often come out in the daytime, so although I would like to have seen them, I hoped at the same time that they would decide to remain nocturnal. I didn't fancy meeting a lion on my own! A few miles outside Biu town, I was also told, there was a volcanic lake, Lake Tilla, where there were crocodiles which were considered to be sacred. The lake was said to harbour no fish, so that nobody seemed to know what the crocodiles fed on. Perhaps they ate all the fish before mere humans could get any. Once a year, I was informed, two goats were sacrificed to keep the crocs happy. However, as they seemed to have taken a couple of goats from the nearby village off their own bat the week before I arrived, I think they were well capable of solving their food requirements themselves.

The main road to Biu, though not tarred, was not bad going on the whole, though I told my parents that it took me about four hours to travel about the distance. However, for driving over laterite roads with lots of potholes and sunken culverts (due to the passage of heavily laden cotton lorries), that was quite a good speed. The smaller roads over which I had to drive in order to reach outlying villages were a different matter – some of them I said in letters home, were like the stony beds of particularly rocky rivers, and had to be seen to be believed. One in fact was indeed a dry riverbed, so that one could only get (by car) to the village in question during the dry season. In the rains, the village was totally cut off from everywhere else. A lot of the road from Maiduguri to Biu, apart from the laterite stretches mentioned above, was, when it went over rocky hills and escarpments, rather like driving up and down a flint staircase. I was very thankful not to have any punctured tyres on that trip. Although I had taken both a camera and cine-camera with me, I was disappointed not to be able to do justice to the magnificent scenery on the journey. The air was still thick with the dust of Harmattan so that what should have been wonderful views was obscured by the haze.

When I reached Biu town, I found that the little bush rest house was high up on the edge of a bluff overlooking a lovely valley. The outlook was superb. The rest house consisted of two small stone buildings, each comprising two tiny rooms, one of which was empty, presumably so that your camp bed could be put there; and the other contained a small table and a couple of dining chairs. There was a small BG off one room. BG stood for *bayan gida* which meant 'behind the house' and was the latrine, which out here in bush was the old thunderbox. We were very sophisticated in Maiduguri on the GRA, having proper flushing loos with septic tank drainage.

125

There was a communal 'kitchen' with the usual wood stove for the cooks to use, and there were boys' quarters nearby. On arrival, Ali and I off-loaded the car and set up 'home'. I was both amused and quite touched to see that Ali, determined that I should conform to the standards that he expected of me in station, had packed my best crockery – also table napkins and even my silver napkin ring! The honour of the doctor was to be firmly upheld. By that time it was getting on in the afternoon, and tired after the hot journey I stretched out on my bed for a siesta. Ali, meantime, set up my camp bath and washbasin in the 'dining room', and started to heat water in the usual bucket on the stove, so that as soon as I surfaced I could wash off the layers of red dust which had enveloped us as we drove along.

I was sitting out on the step a bit later, gazing at the beauty of the valley below me when I heard somebody greeting me. Turning round, I saw coming towards me from the other little rest house, the Provincial Education Officer for Bornu. He was also on tour, to inspect schools in the area. He had only arrived very recently in Maiduguri, having been posted in to take over from the previous PEO who was going on leave. I had met him briefly at various drinks or dinner parties when he was being welcomed to the station, but didn't know him at anything more than that sort of level. Still, it was nice to see a friendly and slightly familiar face. "Are you settled in?" he asked, and went on, "Would you like to share the evening meal with me – I got here yesterday and I rather think my cook bought up the last of the potatoes in the market here. You are welcome to help me eat them." So we shared our meals at the end of each of the days that we were both in Biu, except for one evening when John Bowen, the District Officer (Biu) invited us round to his house for dinner.

The District Officer's house was wonderfully sited, also on the top of the escarpment and overlooking the length of the valley below. For once, I remember, the sky was very clear and the haze seemed to have gone for a time. It was full moon, and the whole valley shone silver as we sat out on the verandah drinking our coffee after the meal. It was unbelievably beautiful and I have never forgotten that evening. John Bowen was later to tease us by saying that he had laid on the full moon specially for the occasion and that it had produced the desired effect – for Rex Abraham (the PEO) and I seemed to hit it off right from the start, and six months later we married.

In the meantime there was still work to be done in Biu Province. Rex carried on with his visits to bush schools, returning to Maiduguri before I did, while I continued my visits to and inspections of, bush dispensaries. En route to nearly all of these, as I mentioned earlier, I would be waved down by people waiting on the roadside who had heard that I would be passing and who brought family members or other people from their villages who were not well so that I could see them on the road.

I also managed to fit in a visit to Garkida in Adamawa Province, farther south, and was shown the mission hospital there – a courtesy visit, but one which I found very interesting. On the way there, incidentally, the car was flagged down by two Fulani warriors. They were two young men, all done up like dandies with colourful make-up on their faces, colourful dress, and carrying spears and clubs and wearing their best jewellery – quite the most exotic chaps I had yet come across. When they halted us, Ali told me to stay in the car while he spoke to them. Then he came back to me and said, "It is all right, Madam, they are just asking if they could be given a lift to Garkida where they are going to see friends." I hoped he'd got it right, but he had. The two young men got into the back seats of the car, folding themselves (they were quite tall) and their weapons carefully in so as not to scratch the upholstery. They sat quietly as I drove along, and when I dropped them off, they thanked me very courteously before going on their way.

As well as attending the dispensaries, I also visited schools to see what the health of the children seemed to be like. They looked like sets of little ragamuffins often, in all kinds of garments, some in shirts and shorts, others in tattered caftans, and yet others in raggedy shirts that barely covered them. They were all excited to see a visitor, and in several schools they paraded proudly in single file out of the main door, round the outside of the building and back in again to their classrooms – all for my benefit. The *Mallam* (the teacher) would bring several children to me that he thought were not too well, so that I could examine them and advise. Most of them, I suggested, should be seen by the dispensary attendant at the nearest dispensary, and I left notes about each with suggestions for treatment to be given when they got there. At one or two villages I was given an 'official' welcome by the District Head, who would come out with all his senior advisers to greet me outside the village walls before I was escorted in through the gateway.

At another village I was taken to meet the chief in his house before being conducted to the dispensary. All this made good sense. The district heads needed to know who was in their territory, just as the British Resident needed to know who was in station. In any case, it was courtesy to make oneself known before diving into work, and courtesy for the local people to welcome visitors. It was also quite an event in some of the outlying places to have anyone go there anyway, and they made the most of it. Why not?

Just before I left one village, the district head sent a messenger to me with the gift of a chicken – a live one of course. In exchange I gave the bearer a 'dash' of money of equal value. I had been advised on first arriving in Nigeria always to offer appropriate recompense for incidental gifts, thus making clear that I was not part of the general 'patronage' culture and therefore under no obligation to anybody. This was understood by the Africans although some would still try to offer that sort of 'gift'. Ali and I put the chicken into the luggage space in the back of my estate car, and anchored it as well as we could to the spare wheel there so that it would not fly all over the car as I drove back to Biu town.

At one point during the journey, there was a lot of noisy clucking and flapping, but I kept on driving and thought to myself 'If it thinks it is going to hop around the car, it is going to be disappointed. Bad luck, chicken.' But when we got back to the rest house, I found to my amusement that it had laid an egg for me, safely into the hollow in the centre of the spare wheel! Two for the price of one, you might say, and certainly an explanation of all the clucking.

When I got back to the little rest house one day, after a visit to a village called Shani, I discovered that my petrol cap was missing. I wasn't surprised, for Shani was totally cut off from everywhere else by road, and the only way that one could get there by car was by driving along a dry riverbed. No vehicle ever went there in the rainy season. The riverbed was pretty uneven with stones and rocks and deep potholes which one tried to avoid and many of which shook the car something chronic. Small wonder that a petrol cap with a slightly dodgy locking device fell off somewhere along the line. Oh well, I thought as I tied a rag round the petrol feed entry, I'll have to find a replacement somehow – probably by buying one in the market – possibly it might even be the one I'd lost, picked up and sold on. One learnt to be philosophical about things in Nigeria, and I got on with the touring. But late in the afternoon of the day following my loss, the Native Authority Health Representative in Biu came to see me. "Doctor, we think this to be yours," he said, proffering a shiny chrome petrol cap. Indeed it was mine – it fitted perfectly, screwed on, and locked. Then he gave me a letter. It was from the Chief of Shani, and had been written for him by the dispensary attendant. The chief had signed it, but being unable to read or write otherwise, had not been able to write himself. It went as follows:

'Shani Dispensary
Biu Division
5th March 58
The Medical Officer Maiduguri
On tour of Biu Division

Madam,
I am directed by the Chief of Shani to write and send you this cover of petrol tank which we thought it to be yours. It was found and brought

to him by a passer on the road of Shani to Buma a distance of 12 miles from Shani.

I hope you would be please to see this and also thank him too. Please write and inform him that you get it safe and it is yours. I think you have reached safely on that day.

Yours obedient servant

Othman Kadafur. Dispensary attendant, Shani

Countersigned by

Adama Sarkin Shani [Chief of Shani]'

I asked where the messenger was, so that I could thank him and give him a suitable reward. 'Oh, he has already gone,' said the Health Representative, 'He was told by the chief that he was not to stop at all on the way here because they did not know how long you would remain in Biu, and he was also told to return to Shani immediately and report back to the chief. Now Shani was a lot of miles out of Biu town so far as I recall. The man had walked the whole distance, and had set out to return without even stopping for a rest. He had travelled right through the night, I was told, over rough, hilly and probably hyena infested country, so as to reach me before I left. He didn't own a horse and had no bicycle, so that it had to be walking or nothing. I left some money and a letter with John Bowen, the District Officer, so that when he next went to Shani, which he said he would be doing shortly, he could deliver them appropriately for me.

"How did they know the petrol cap would be mine?" I asked the Health Officer. He replied, "The people all know that if anybody finds anything unusual they must always take it to the chief who would then decide what if anything was to be done. That way nobody can ever be accused of stealing anything, everybody is honest, and the chief knows exactly what is going on in his area. Nobody else had driven that way for some months, so the petrol cover had to be yours." I still have the letter, and I still marvel at the whole event.

While in Biu I made an effort to visit Lake Tilla, hoping to see the crocodiles there. I set off for the lake before breakfast and before my official day's touring. It was really quite beautiful – the blue colours of the water and sky complementing one another, and interest being added by the presence of women from the nearby village doing their laundry by beating it all on large flat stones which were just under the water surface. First of all they would spread everything out on the stones and then rub soap all over it. After that, whatever was being washed was folded over, still on the stones, and beaten hard for several minutes to work the soap in. After that it was unfolded and rinsed in deeper water before being taken back to the village and spread out on the ground to dry. It would all have dried in a matter of minutes – no need for spin driers in that climate! So there was plenty going on for me to see and take in. But crocodiles? Where were they? Ali, who had come along with me, and I, wandered round to a part of the lake where there were no other people thrashing about at the water's edge. We waited. And waited. And then – the head of a crocodile broke the surface of the lake not far away from us. It turned this way and that, inspecting its surroundings. It came up a bit more and then – had it seen me and taken fright at the sight? – precipitately sank, never to reappear. And that was all I ever saw of the Lake Tilla crocodiles.

Well, after all the bush schools had been inspected and the children medically examined, and after all the bush dispensaries had been checked likewise, records looked at, medicines sorted out, injection licences verified, all the various courtesy visits made, it was time to return to Maiduguri.

Biu had been a lovely area to go to, and the rest house had been a good place to stay in, sited as it was above that beautiful valley. The journey between Biu and Maiduguri was also full of interest in spite of the rough dusty roads. En route I'd seen baboons, small monkeys, and the odd antelope – all bounding along ahead of me. The red dust was something you had to experience in order to believe – when I finally got home I was covered with it from top to toe, as was the car and all my loads, and as was Ali. I told my parents that despite the road surfaces, I'd done the journey in less than four hours. And that, for nearly fifty years ago, I reckon was quite good going.

I commented also in my letter home that it made a difference not having other traffic to contend with – I'd probably not seen another vehicle, or at the most, the odd lorry carrying cotton in all that distance. These lorries, incidentally, were very heavy and gouged out great lots of sand from the road surface, so that, especially at culverts, you would suddenly find yourself coming to a sudden halt in one of the hollows they left.

One learnt all sorts of driving techniques out there that one never knew existed!

Chapter 17

Things got back to normal in Maiduguri in that for a brief spell both Louis and I were there and we could get on with 'big' theatre cases that had been waiting for us both. We were always busy. At this time too, we had expected a smallpox outbreak. However, luckily for our area we only had a few cases, and as the time slipped by, the likelihood of any more diminished for that year at least, we hoped. But we did have at the same time many cases of chicken pox and measles. At first I had found it difficult to make out a measles rash on a dark skin, but it wasn't long before it was quite easy for me to diagnose – one soon 'acclimatised' to the different appearances.

By now – mid March – it was getting a lot hotter. Biu had been cooler than Maiduguri anyway, so that I noticed the difference when I got back into station.

In a letter home I now wrote 'I am sleeping on top of the bed with nothing on but the fan' and said how I would wake and get up at about 2 a.m. and have a cold bath to try to cool down. However, I added that the water came warmish out of the cold tap so that it didn't really help a lot.

I was quite pleased one day to realise that Amadu, my teenage 'small boy' had begun to speak to me only in Hausa. Hitherto he had always used what English he had (quite a lot actually). Now he had decided that as I was taking lessons, and as he had heard on the grapevine that I was speaking as much as I could in my pidgin Hausa to patients at the hospital, it was time for him to extend my linguistic education. He began by speaking slowly to me, and correcting me when I got things wrong. When I got it right, then like a good teacher he encouraged and congratulated me. I felt that this was a big compliment and was quite touched. At the hospital, the patients did seem to appreciate the fact that to a certain extent they could speak to me directly instead of through a nurse. It did wonders for my ego, and though I am sure that much of what I was picking up would be the idiom of the market place, did that matter? I was communicating.

During the Hot Season, I discovered an unexpected pleasure, albeit a very slight one. Probably I've said earlier that one didn't, or I didn't, try to put make-up on because it simply melted and ran off. But I would generally still put on a dash of lipstick if I was invited out in the evening when it was a little bit cooler. One had to keep lipstick (and other makeup if used) in the fridge, otherwise it melted into a slushy treacly mess. Now it was a tiny bit of luxury when dressing for dinner, to get the lovely cold lipstick out and put some on, even if the sensation was only momentary.

As I write this memoir, recollections drift through my mind, some unbidden, others summoned up when I read through letters that I sent home all those years ago. In one such letter (March 1958) I mentioned anthropologists, several of whom passed through Maiduguri from time to time, or set up camp not very far away. To some extent, people viewed what they did with some scepticism, as it was felt that they came for relatively short times, asked lots of questions of the locals, and then departed without a backward glance to write their books. Probably that was not all true, but it was a feeling strongly expressed to me when I was there. What is more, many of them on arrival immediately got themselves into native dress, doubtless feeling that this was a good integrating thing to do. In fact at that time, many of the indigenous people didn't really approve of that. Native costume was something that was presented as a formal and rather special gift to expatriates who were leaving – and often only if they were leaving on retirement at that. I don't think just being posted to another station generally warranted such a gift. So I think local people felt it a bit presumptive for expatriates to adopt native dress almost on arrival. I could be wrong and stand to be corrected, but that was certainly my impression then.

I do remember, and indeed told in a letter home, that a couple of anthropologists who had visited some time before my arrival in Nigeria and who were said to be very earnest in their investigations, had been taken for a ride by the villagers. We heard this from some of the locals who came through to the hospital outpatient clinic. The village, it seems, en masse had decided that these two were a bit crazy, so thought it would be fun to string them along. Accordingly the men had made up all sorts of stories about their shaving customs, all of which had been duly recorded by the two investigators. The villagers, they told us, had a good laugh, and presumably the anthropologists had a feeling of satisfaction at what they had discovered. I pass on this anecdote for what it is worth – it certainly came to me from 'sources' which I considered to be reliable. What did rather needle me was the fact that from time to time, anthropologists who set up home in local villages, trying to 'live as the people did', would then come to us in a panic saying that they thought they had contracted all kinds of diseases and demanding instant treatment. These were supposedly intelligent men and women who surely knew about simple health and hygiene measures when they came out. Why on earth did they simply ignore what they had learnt? It only put an extra burden on the hard worked health staff, who had plenty to do without having to look after irresponsible men and women like that.

I have already mentioned the fact that patients often handed me letters on first attending the clinic – letters written either by themselves or by scribes

132

on their behalf. Either way, it made for some very odd missives. In particular, one stands out – and indeed I still have that letter among my papers. The letter, after going into long reams of information which told me nothing about the actual symptoms, but which asked for lots of treatment, finished up with the sentence:

"I hope your doctorship will grant this my humble request."

I had never been called 'my doctorship' before. It made me feel quite important.

It is wrong to laugh at things like this, for I know that the poor soul in question was trying to get help, but I probably made much funnier attempts to say things in Hausa for which I would expect to be chuckled at – indeed this happened more than once. Sometimes elaborate letters were written in order to try to get preferential treatment. This never cut any ice with either Louis or me. Everyone took their turn unless it was clearly something very urgent. Often women would have letters written for them by their husbands, which they would silently hand to me and then wait for a magic pronouncement. On the whole, letters seemed to be written only by Southern Nigerians. The Hausa people didn't go for self referral in the same way – they spoke up for themselves as soon as seen.

Some of the most common complaints were 'fever and pains all over' (which usually meant malaria), and 'ciwon sanyi', which meant gonorrhoea. It can rightly be said that venereal disease is not a respecter of people, but I think that from what I saw, it was better to say that the people I was seeing, no matter who they were, from the highest to the lowest, were no respecters of venereal disease.

As students at medical school, we were told in our VD lectures that 'The male is the indicator'. Judging from the number of cases of gonorrhoea among the men that came to the clinics, there must have been far more women in Northern Nigeria similarly infected than ever came to me for treatment. No wonder it was rife. And remembering that, I am not at all surprised at the present decimating spread of AIDS in Sub-Saharan Africa.

Well, I'd got back from tour and was once again enveloped in hospital work. Louis had to go to Kano for a few days, after which we planned to get through a lot of theatre work before I went off to bush again. To our irritation we had to delay things for a time because of an official visit to Maiduguri by the Permanent Secretary to the Ministry of Health. Eventually we got through everything and once again Ali and I packed up the car and off we went, this time north to Gashua and Nguru.

Louis had warned me that some of the roads I'd have to use to get to outlying dispensaries in that area were impassable by ordinary cars. He therefore had arranged for me to be taken in our hospital Land Rover. However, at the last moment the Land Rover broke down and was firmly out of commission, so I had to set off in my own car after all, and hoped to be able to organise some alternative form of transport at the other end. Accompanying me were Ali, my stalwart cook-major-domo, and the Maiduguri Native Authority Health Representative. It was Ramadan at the time of this journey – the month of fasting between sunrise and sunset. I had been given to understand that Moslems were allowed to break the fast in the event of illness or long journeys, so long as they 'paid back' a day at the end of the month for each day of broken fasting. However, neither of my two passengers would break their fast, which made me feel very awkward when I had to stop the car in order to have a drink. We had taken flasks of water and squash with us, and I knew that I needed the fluid. I had to be able to drive safely and could not risk becoming drowsy or otherwise affected by the heat and dehydration. I reminded myself that both the men were well accustomed to the heat, had survived many years of Ramadan fasting, and they both knew what they were doing.

The road became more and more sandy the farther north we got, and in the end it was very deep soft sand and driving through it was not easy. The best way I can describe it is by suggesting that it was a bit like trying to drive through deep soft snow in an ordinary car without wheel chains. Anyway, eventually we reached Gashua after a long and tiring journey. I decided that the best place to go to in order to ask about possible transport was the local Native Authority Police HQ. I was to stay that night in Nguru with the District Officer and his wife there, so I needed an immediate means of getting there. Louis had already told me that when I left my car in Gashua, I should ask permission to leave it at this HQ which should ensure that it was safe from thieves. Nguru was another forty miles along the road.

The only thing anyone could come up with was a lorry which, I told my parents later, I was sure had never in its long life seen either springs or shock absorbers. I was told it was sometimes used as a refuse cart. In it we travelled to Nguru, did a round trip of 80 miles to bush dispensaries the next day as well as the return trip of 40 miles back to Gashua. Ali and our loads were hefted into the back of the lorry while the Health Representative and I travelled in the cab with the driver.

The driver and Health Rep decided that I should sit between them in the middle (ostensibly so that I should not be in any danger of falling out en route, the passenger door not being too secure). This meant that I hadn't too much room for my feet as the foot wells were on either side but there was no space in the middle. Talk about an uncomfortable and bone crushing means of travelling – I felt as if I'd been crippled for life when I struggled out of that

134

lorry each time, especially when I knew I would have to get into it again for further journeys! As the Health Rep was a tall man, I could hardly suggest that he changed places with me another time, so I just had to put up with it.

I was very glad to reach the District Officer's house in Nguru at the end of that first day, where I could bath and get rid of the sand which covered me, and drink lots of long cool drinks – I must have run their water supplies almost dry within the first five minutes. I had not realised just how dehydrated I must have been until I reached out my hand to start one drink and found that the glass was already empty – I must have downed it straight off without even knowing. Even worse – the D.O. and his wife told me that Tom Letchworth, the Resident for Bornu, was also on tour in Nguru and would be coming to join us for dinner that night. I hadn't exactly packed my best going-out-for-dinner dress with me, not expecting such a formal event far out in bush country, but I did my best with what I'd got. We had a very pleasant evening, and of course I'd met Tom Letchworth in Maiduguri so it wasn't as if he was a stranger. However, I was far too tired by that time to take much part in the conversation. I rather think I'd had to put in two or three hours at the hospital before even leaving Maiduguri that day – and after the meal when we were having coffee, I kept falling asleep out of sheer exhaustion and finally had to excuse myself and go to bed. The D.O. reprimanded me a bit the next morning. "Never go to sleep in front of the Resident," he told me, "You have to keep awake and go on talking." But Tom had not been offended, and had seen how done I was.

The next day was taken up with a long round trip to outlying villages and dispensaries, finishing up with the journey back to Gashua. Here I settled into the little bush rest house. It consisted of just one room with a tiny washroom and thunderbox loo off it. There was a big mesh cage built outside, separate from the rest house but only a yard or two away, where, in the hot season, one set up one's camp bed. It being the hot season now, I put my bed there. After my evening meal and a short time reading a library book, I turned in, locking the cage door against thieves and tucking myself under my mosquito net. I soon slept. Some time later on I was rudely woken by an unearthly animal sound, not quite a roar and not quite a shriek, but whatever it was, it was not far away. Suddenly the mesh of the cage looked very fragile. I felt, and was, totally alone, and the breeze blocks of the rest house seemed inviting and safe. I listened again, and suddenly the sound came once more, seeming really very near. That decided me, and I quietly unlocked the cage door and that of the rest house, and then in one mad movement I pulled the camp bed, poles, net and all, from the cage and into the rest house. I kicked myself for being such a coward, but at least I felt safe again inside solid walls, and slept like a log until morning. I wondered if I had heard hyenas, which

I had been told roamed about the town at night. Alone and rather isolated from other people, I had been one very nervous medical officer! Everything seemed different the next morning when it was light.

One of my forays on that tour was to a little almost forgotten town – Gorgoram. At one time it had been the administrative headquarters for that general area. The Emir had lived there and all the Native Authority executive officers had been there too. Then everything was moved elsewhere and the Emir now lived in Gashua. Gorgoram fell into disuse and most of its inhabitants moved out. Once again I had to travel in the springless, shock absorberless lorry.

To get to Gorgoram we travelled through what seemed to be totally trackless bush. No signs of life anywhere. I decided that instead of using signposts, one had to think something like 'Turn off at the third tree on the left, carry on for a bit and then turn right at the clump of thornbush with an old tree trunk just behind it.' What would happen if any trees were to be felled, I wondered. I felt as if I was being taken to the ends of the earth and asked myself if we would ever find our way back. However, the driver seemed to know what he was doing.

Finally we rattled over a patch of very bumpy lumpy ground that I guessed could be all swamp in the rainy season, and there, in front of me, were the remnants of the mud wall which had surrounded a once thriving little town. Only about ten people still lived there, and they all turned out to welcome me as we drove through the disintegrating gateway. Most of the bigger buildings had fallen down and were crumbling away, only a few small mud houses remaining. The tiny bush dispensary was housed in the only big building still standing. Originally this building had housed the local Treasury.

I would have been one of the last Government officials to go there to do a formal inspection, for I was told that the dispensary too was shortly being closed down and was moving to a bigger centre. Looking at this little lost town, I had a strong impression of past splendours now lost in the present shadows. It was a pathetic sight and I felt sad to see how totally the mud buildings had fallen away and were now not much more than dust, which in its turn would merge with the sandy foundations on which they had all been built. Already the bush was encroaching on the outskirts, and soon would take over altogether. I found myself thinking of the impermanence and smallness of mankind and of the power of Nature.

For the moment however, I was made very welcome, and conducted a little clinic for the few people still there, before doing a final inspection of the medicines and records. No point here, I thought, on reporting the maintenance of the buildings.

It was while I was based in Gashua that I invented shandy. Don't tell

136

me that shandy had been around since time immemorial – I know. But at that time, not being a beer drinker – or indeed, much of a drinker at all other than a drinker of squash, I had not heard of shandy. This particular day, after hours of being shaken around in that lorry, and after having been gasping for a long drink all the way back to the rest house, for some strange reason I could think of nothing but having some beer. I had no idea what it would taste like, but I knew that I wanted some. As soon as I got back to my little temporary home, I asked Ali if he could get me a bottle of beer from somewhere. Diplomatically, he made no comment, simply saying, "Yes, Madam," but I sensed his surprise as he went off. He returned a little later with a bottle of Star beer. 'Ah! Star!' said the advertisements for it, and indeed I felt as if I wore the same expression of thankful delight as the man on the posters. I poured out a glassful and drank. Yes, it was like I had imagined, but I wanted a bit more sweetness. I made up half a glass of squash and topped it up with the beer (lager, really, it was), and bingo! I had invented the most delicious shandy. I've never tasted a better one since. The bottle was soon empty and my dehydration cured.

My last visit on that tour was to another outlying dispensary. The attendant there was a very intelligent man who was extremely interested in his work. Unlike many of the others, he was licensed to give several different kinds of injections. He could treat bilharzia which needed one kind of injection, and he was also allowed to give injections of penicillin for other complaints. He had used his skills wisely, only giving that antibiotic when he felt it to be really necessary. Most patients, I should point out, demanded injections, which they thought were more powerful than oral medicines, and it was always a temptation for somebody with only a simple training, to give in to these demands. Moreover, he had organised a tiny space in his dispensary that he said was his 'hospital', where I found that he admitted an occasional very sick person, so that he could stay on duty all the time and look after his patient. In this way he had treated several cases of pneumonia during the rainy season, and felt that his use of penicillin for them had been justified. I agreed and thought he had done well.

However, his pièce de résistance had yet to be shown to me. This, also of his own devising, was a 'shower room'. He had built a small unroofed 'room' out of zana matting – a sort of woven grass matting. Inside he had put up a high pole with a hook at the top. On the hook was hung a big zinc bucket. This he had filled with water and left there, so that with evaporation it would cool. A rope attached to it would invert the bucket so that the water tipped out and all over anyone who stood underneath. This was the shower, and he had organised it because some of his patients needed both cleaning up and cooling down, he told me. All this was explained to me through the Health Representative, who interpreted from the rapid Hausa into English for me. "And doctor," added the Health Rep, "he says that nobody has yet been allowed to use it because everyone knew that you were coming. It was decided that you would be the very first person to have a shower, in honour of your visit and to declare it officially open."

I must say, it was the last thing I had expected, miles from anywhere in the depths of the bush. I was sure that if I went into the little grass 'room' and stripped off for a shower, several pairs of eyes would be silently peeping through the spaces in the woven grass. It wouldn't be every day that they had a chance to see what white women looked like under their clothes.

But it was hot, dry and dusty and I was weary after bumping around in that lorry, so I didn't care – into the shower I went and obediently inaugurated it with a sharp pull on the rope, thereupon being deluged with lovely cold water. It was well worth it in spite of possible spying eyes. I imagine that not many people will ever have been asked to 'open' a shower-bath in such a formal manner!

While in Nguru, as part of my duties, I had to inspect the local slaughter slab to see if it was kept clean and decent. It was really only a large concreted area with a channel round the edges for blood to be swilled off to sink into the surrounding sand. The day I went there was in fact one of the killing days. All the butchery had been finished and only various entrails were still lying there. The concrete had not yet been washed down. The slab was occupied by a whole lot of vultures, all looking, as I always thought, like so many black raggedy umbrellas hopping about. They were busily attacking the gory remnants of camels, goats and cattle, and I have to say they were making a pretty good job of it. Clearly it was sensible to leave the slab for the vultures to clean up first before the locals finished off. Water only came from wells, and was a precious commodity. If the vultures took most of the mess away, less water would be needed to complete the job.

Not far away, nearer to the market place, several strings of camels had just arrived in from the desert, and were couched on the sand waiting to be unloaded before, I suppose, being taken to drink. I realised again how near I was to the Sahara. They all looked weary as well as disdainful, and I wondered how far they had come that day.

I also had to inspect the 'dried meat factories'. They were, in fact, small mud buildings within the domestic compounds of their owners (at least the ones I saw were), where strips of meat taken, I suppose, from freshly butchered animals, were laid out in the sun to dry. I think the meat must have been first smoked after a fashion. I am still not sure what I was supposed to do when 'inspecting' them. Anyway, it was interesting, and I recorded that they had been visited and reported that the small establishments appeared to be clean and well looked after.

I was able to do my last visits in my own car at long last, and how good it was not to have to be shaken and bumped about in the lorry! Nevertheless, in spite of the easier going, I had to drive through bush so thick that branches literally poked through the open car windows at times. However, two dispensaries and sixty miles more on the odometer, I had finished everything I had to do. Although I was not expected to return to Maiduguri until the next day, I decided that as it was still only lunch time, I would not sit in the rest house doing nothing for another twenty four hours but would set off and get back home that same day. That should give me a quiet night in a proper bed before being played back in to hospital duties again. Ali and I packed up in record time and were soon on the road. The sand on which I had to drive was very soft and very deep. The middle of the road had been gouged out by the occasional lorries that went over it, so that I felt as if I was slithering along in a narrow gully with high banks on each side of it. Everything was very hot, it being the middle of the day. Suddenly the car seemed to skid along the sand and mounted the banks first on one side and then the other. By some miracle it didn't turn over before I managed to stop. One of my tubeless tyres had blown out. This meant that I had to offload the back of the car in order to get the spare wheel out from its under-floor recess before changing the two wheels over. Everything was so scorching that I could hardly manage to touch anything, and it was quite a problem coping with the metal tools. At least, when one began to drive, the steering wheel, though sizzling at first, cooled down a bit, but tools permanently closed up under the loading area remained just about at boiling point and one was in danger of getting burnt hands from them.

We all carried tubeless tyre repair kits and I was accustomed to dealing with ordinary punctures and changing wheels. But this time my tyre had a big hole in it and was not repairable. I had no second spare, so that if the same thing were to happen again I would be well and truly sunk. I drove very carefully and slowly after that, keeping my fingers crossed, and for once was sorry that there wasn't any traffic for the next hundred miles. In fact I still didn't see any other vehicle for many miles after I had rejoined the main Maiduguri-Jos road later on. I'm not quite sure what I would have done if there had been another blow out. We were not carrying unlimited amounts of water, and goodness knows how long it would have been before anyone realised that I was in trouble. As I said, nobody in Maiduguri was expecting me before the next day, and there would be nobody in Nguru who would know if anything happened to me on the road once I'd left there. Probably the safest thing would have been to stay exactly where we were and to conserve water as much as we could and wait for somebody to pass by – which may have been later that day or not until the next or even the one after that. Anyway, the devil looks after his own, I suppose, and we got home safely without further mishap, Ali and I. I had been lucky.

A week later, the rains broke. How lovely it was. Oddly, there had been no build-up. Normally the transition from dry hot season to the rains was presaged by a few weeks of intensely hot and very humid weather. This time, the day had started off as usual, hot and dry, and then suddenly towards the end of the afternoon, in spite of clear blue sky, there was a crash of thunder and within minutes the heavens opened and the rain teemed down for well over an hour.

My next letter home said:

'5.4.1958

It's extraordinary what a strange smell has come with the rain, the smell I noticed when we first pulled in to the coast of Africa when I was on my way here, I suppose it is the steamy smell of dirt and dry dust and the trees etc, but it came up a few seconds after it began to rain. I can see I shall have to get some gum boots too when I am in Kaduna, as my compound is full of lakes at the moment. I might have guessed there was something on the way as late last night, long after I had gone to bed, there was a sudden wind and the curtains started blowing all over the place which has never happened before.'

I can remember it now, more than fifty years later on. It was the first rain I'd seen for six months.

Not so long after that I was due to go to Kaduna to attend a course on leprosy. I hoped there wouldn't be rain on the journey, as I would be travelling along a dry season road. Such roads, if rain was heavy, would be closed to all travellers, with ordinary cars being made to wait for six hours at the barrier after each storm before being allowed to proceed. Lorries and other heavy vehicles would be held up for twelve hours. There were a lot of barrier points along these roads.

The time came for my trip. The whole journey was about 500 miles, but because of the nature of the roads, Louis had arranged for me to take three days over it. I stopped first at Potiskum about 160 miles on. There the local District Officer invited me to his house for dinner. It was a lonely-ish posting as he was the only European living on the station, and I think he was always glad to have visitors. Although he could in theory drive to Jos quite easily, he would not be able to leave his station exactly every weekend. In any case his duties would take him out to bush, not to the bright lights of Jos. Onwards I went the next day another two hundred miles to Jos, my next stop.

When driving, journeys soon seemed to be so ordinary that one could forget that one was travelling through quite wild country. I certainly did, and it was not until one time when I had stopped the car and nipped several yards from the side of the road to the privacy of some dense thickets and trees in order to answer a call of nature that it was brought home to me. While very much engaged there, there was a sudden heavy crashing and thrashing about just behind me – undoubtedly some large animal had been unceremoniously disturbed by my activities, and (luckily for me) had decided to make itself scarce rather than go into attack mode. I was quite glad to get back to the car, reflecting that Nigerian bush was not exactly your average English copse.

The road except for the last ninety miles of it, was much more dry and dusty than when I had first driven over it several months earlier. This was because now we had just had the dry season, and before that, Harmattan with all its dust as well. There had not yet been much in the way of rain to dampen things down. Finally I set out the next morning on the last lap to Kaduna, coming down off the Jos plateau past tall rocks and hills, eventually driving through forested country. It was a very beautiful road but also very lonely. Generally, even if there was no traffic, you would at least see the odd person walking, perhaps herding a few cows, or riding a donkey. Here I saw nobody, although I had the impression from time to time that somebody had just filtered off the road and into the trees. The only living thing that I saw at all was a great warthog which suddenly dashed out of the trees and across the road right in front of the car. I only just missed it.

On this trip I had no need of my cook Ali, because I was to stay in the Catering Rest House so that all my meals would be taken care of and I would have a good room to myself. Kaduna was the Administrative HQ for Northern Nigeria and was therefore SOPHISTICATED. I hoped that there would be some decent canteens and stores from where I could stock up with a few luxuries. Alas, Kaduna had very little in the way of canteens. Jos was far better. However, it was sensible to have somebody with me who could speak Hausa properly, in case of road problems, so I took my small boy Amadu with me instead. Amadu was very thrilled to be coming to Kaduna, especially as the trip was to be a real holiday for him. I would not need looking after, so all he had to do was to keep in contact with me every day and to be ready to travel back home at the right time. Otherwise his time would be his own, and as he was able to stay in boys' quarters by the Rest House, I knew he would be all right.

In Jos he was very excited because for the first time in his life he saw a railway and a train – things he had only heard of until then. And when we arrived in Kaduna, he was deeply impressed and said to me, "This plenty big town, madam." He looked again and said, "Maiduguri be very bush town Madam."

As usual, anyone who went out of station to a bigger centre had a very long shopping list because friends and neighbours all wanted things getting for them. I was no exception. But Kaduna was really rather disappointing from the point of view of those exciting little extras like stuffed olives. However I did manage to get a few lengths of cotton material to make up and replenish my dwindling supply of dresses skirts and blouses all of which had started to disintegrate with the effects of sun and sweat. But when I tried to buy some light shoes and sandals I was told, "We don't stock large sizes Madam." I felt a bit like a monster from outer space at that!

One item I was rather amused to find in Kaduna (I wasn't looking for it but just happened to see it) was a supply of Allinson's Whole Wheat Flour. Normally in Maiduguri, Ali would buy flour in the market, for he made bread every day. You didn't buy loaves there as we do here. Only once, years later, in Maiduguri, I saw a little handcart being trundled round the streets. It was built like a glass sided cupboard on wheels. It was full of loaves of bread, and on the outside of it were the words 'Buy Olympic Charlie bread for decency and strength'. Marvellous. I couldn't resist buying some Allinson's, for my father in his retirement had taken to baking as something to do, and prided himself on his breadmaking, using that flour. I told Ali that if he could make as good bread with it as my father did, I would judge him a really superlative cook. And of course he did, for he was superlative anyway.

While I was in Kaduna the rains broke there and I thrilled to the many wonderful tropical storms we had. They are so dramatic and exhilarating and the whole world seems to crackle and spark with extra life while they are on.

On the return journey to Maiduguri the roads were quite different following that few days of rain. Now there were waterholes all along the way at which herds of cattle were drinking. Normally they would have to wait for water to be given to them in turn in big calabashes drawn from deep wells.

The Leprosy lectures were interesting as were the visits to Leprosy clinics and hospitals. It had been a very useful week, even though in Maiduguri I only ever needed to refer Leprosy cases to the Mission doctor at Molai. And yes, in case you were wondering, I found most of the commodities in Jos that I couldn't get hold of in Kaduna, so I was a popular person when I got back home as I went round like Santa Claus, delivering goodies to all and sundry.

On the way home, Amadu was telling me about the things he had done in Kaduna, which chiefly consisted of wandering round to see everything there. I think some of the Rest House boys had taken him under their wing and looked after him a bit. However, he said to me that Kaduna was very expensive. I had already given him extra money with which to look after himself there, and I feared that perhaps I hadn't given him enough. His normal pay was fifteen shillings weekly and he got his living quarters as well. I asked him how much it had cost him for his food in Kaduna. He told me that he had spent about eight shillings on food there.

"How much does it cost you in Maiduguri, then?" I asked him.

"Only five shillings," he replied.

Amadu was a healthy well fed looking youngster who was obviously getting enough to eat in Maiduguri. It was interesting to know what it cost the boys to keep themselves. They didn't have to pay anything for their quarters, and they had several sets of uniform provided for their working day so that they didn't have to spend too much on clothes. I had worried a bit about their pay when I first went out, but realised from what Amadu now told me that he was really well satisfied with what he got. He had plenty of friends who visited him, and he seemed to buy himself little luxuries of his own as and when he wanted them, so I stopped worrying.

Once back home with the rains having broken well and truly, I engaged a garden boy. In the dry season there had not been really anything to do in the compound, but now everything began to grow. The coarse grass seemed to get taller even as you looked at it. We were all supposed to keep our own compounds tidy and free from places where mosquitoes could breed, so now would be a busy time.

The garden boy certainly made the place look a lot more orderly and he worked quite hard. One day I found that there were a lot of plants growing where there had been a bare patch the day before. I fondly thought the boy had been growing them somewhere at the back from seed and had just planted them out. But – "Your garden boy was round at my house," said Louis to me with a twinkle, "Begging plants from my garden. He told my boy that you needed them." I was horrified. "Louis, I said no such thing!" "Don't worry, girl," replied Louis, "I knew perfectly well you would never do that. But I said he could have them just the same." And he laughed.

I was much amused one day when, having just arrived for work, my garden boy had to take cover from a huge rainstorm before he could even start. In seconds the compound was awash. When the rain eventually stopped, I could hardly believe my eyes when the boy came out again and solemnly began to water all the plants, for that was part of his duties and he had clearly intended to do it first.

Only in Africa!

The rains continued, and in between downpours everything was very hot and humid. I never seemed to dry out but constantly dripped with – not ladylike perspiration – but good old-fashioned SWEAT. I drank more squash than I'd ever done, yet the liquid streaming from my pores seemed to leave me feeling just as thirsty as ever. Despite this and the inevitable prickly heat I was not really uncomfortable – it all seemed to be a normal part of life.

Ali, my cook, was worth his weight in gold. Everyone envied me having Ali, especially as I was known for my small appetite. If I was entertaining, Ali was always the star of the event. Once, I had arranged a pre-Open Night drinks party, and just as Ali and I had started between us to prepare the food for it, I was (inevitably) called down to the hospital. When I finally got back home just as the first guests arrived, it was to find that Ali had everything organised. The food was all ready and beautifully presented, the drinks and bottled water were all cool. Everything was point device, and Ali himself, imperturbable as ever was there in a spotlessly white uniform, all ready to serve drinks and hand round plates of food. It was like having a fairy godmother in the house.

Louis decided at the last minute to try to do one final tour round part of the province before the ever increasing rains washed some of the roads out for three months. Already the local plane service was occasionally disrupted because of storms. These tropical storms, though exhilarating to watch, particularly with the startling and brilliant lightning flashes, could be violent and could do considerable damage.

I have said that the MO left in station at such times was pretty busy. This was not only because of the added clinical workload but because of the administration too. I only had to tackle that when Louis was out of station, and even then I only had to attend to part of it – the rest could wait till his return – but what I did was enough to make me realise just what a lot of work was involved in the running of the hospital. The office work was tedious as much as anything. Absolutely everything in the way of admin had to be covered by the MO in charge, from the simplest things like ordering, or authorising orders for, soaps, linen, foods and so on, to the more complicated matters of seeing to the leave requirements for hospital staff. Matron would deal with that sort of thing in respect of nursing staff, though Louis would have to approve, but there were many other members of staff too – the cooks, labourers, drivers, messengers, gatekeepers, night watchmen and many others. And there was always the pharmacy order to contend with when everything else was done.

Many of the hospital employees were not paid monthly as we ourselves were, and did not receive salary direct from Kaduna. There were weekly paid staff, daily paid staff, even a few hourly paid staff. Making all these payments could be very time consuming, especially as the safe could only be opened if both the MO in charge and the chief clerk were present with their two keys at the same time. Because of the ever present dangers of corruption, nothing was ever left unlocked, however much one trusted members of staff. Not everyone was corrupt by any means, but you never really knew who was and who was not, with only a few exceptions. Payments for many members of staff had to be made in cash because hardly any would have bank accounts. We ourselves simply had pay slips sent to us and our salaries paid directly into our banks, but most of our African staff would not be the same.

My practice when on my own at the hospital was to try to clear the desk twice each morning – once just before I started the outpatient clinics, and once after these clinics were finished and before I started on my ward rounds and theatre work.

Then, at the end of each morning, and once I had attended to the bulk of the clinical work (but always before the chief clerk went off duty at 2 p.m.), I would clear the desk for a final time for that day. The desk always seemed to be piled high with files for the MO to attend to – no sooner had you reached the bottom of one pile than the next began to accumulate, or so it seemed. But it was all good experience.

Connected with the job, but this time on the social side, it was always a pleasant duty to have to entertain very senior people from Kaduna when they came round the province to see how things were getting on. 'Kaduna' was not just the name of the headquarters town, it was the name given by everyone to the Government departments collectively. 'What does Kaduna say?' or 'Have you asked Kaduna?' were common questions amongst senior staff. Alternatively, you would be told 'I'll write to Kaduna about it' if some particular problem had arisen.

Government administration was steered very much by 'General Orders' – in other words, we operated strictly by the book. Every possible permutation and combination of circumstance seemed to be dealt with in the General Orders Book, and everyone knew that if in any doubt, all one had to do was to refer to General Orders and there one would find the answer. If at times this all seemed to be rather rigid, it was nevertheless a very practical arrangement because one always knew where one stood. Highly confidential letters, for instance, should only be typed and sent by heads of department or, on occasions, other senior service officers. Clerks were not to be involved. The General Orders book made this clear, even to telling what colour typing should be used, and instructing that such letters should first be sealed in an envelope, then sealed into a second envelope before being dispatched – where to? – 'To Kaduna' of course. General Orders provided both a source of amusement to us all but also a firm support for which many were very thankful.

Somehow in amongst my official duties I managed to find time to do

145

some dressmaking, and soon had a few garments put together to replace those which were now disintegrating rapidly. The Club librarian had recently managed to make an arrangement (through Singer's) to have a Butterick pattern book sent for the library each month. We could then order patterns from it via Singer's in Lagos, and with luck, our orders would arrive two or three weeks later on. Half of us, needless to say, chose the same styles to make up, but what did that matter? We had generally bought different materials so we didn't look all identical. Certainly I didn't look identical to anyone else, as although I was a good kid with surgical sutures, I was hopeless with dressmaking, and had to settle for wearing dresses which at most covered me decently but didn't do much more for me. Trimmings, braids, buttons, hooks and eyes, elastic, bra repair outfits and so on were usually difficult to get locally, and I had almost a standing order with my mother to send me supplies of things like that, for which I was more than grateful.

As the rains came to an end, the temperature rose. At least with a rainstorm, although it was extremely humid, things were a little cooler for a short time. The day came when I wrote to my parents:

'19.5.1958

It's amazing, I have just been to get myself a drink, and the glass feels warm as I pick it up. This morning when I got up, I was picking up my torch which I keep under the pillow, as my switch doesn't always work for the bedhead light. The torch is a metal one and it was almost too hot to hold! And my dress which had been hanging over the rail all night, in the draught from the fan and the windows (it was a bit windy last night) felt when I put it on as if I had just taken it out of the hot airing cupboard. Can you imagine that?

...I just can't imagine what I shall be like when I get home, I shall take to hot water bottles, I expect! That will be a blow to my pride! This letter seems to harp on the heat, but it is interesting to me to see how I have adapted myself to it, and it is all so different from anything at home that I am trying to get it across to you.'

Chapter 18

Other, more personal matters were occupying my mind by this time as well as the medical work. The new PEO, Rex Abraham and I, when we met at the Biu Rest House and shared a few meals there, had got on together very well, discovering that we had a great deal in common, both in our backgrounds, and also in the way in which we thought about many issues. On return to station we continued to see one another and a strong friendship developed which, before long, we both realised was becoming something much deeper and more serious, and we were spending more and more time together. It appeared that unknown to us, the rest of the station was observing us closely. Indeed, although we only found out much later on, from then on each time either of us hosted a party, the station made up its mind that this would be an engagement party.

We had known each other for about a couple of months when Rex suddenly had to go back to the UK on compassionate leave as his father was very ill. At first he didn't know if he would ever be able to return to Nigeria, but things improved, and eventually his plane touched down once more at the Maiduguri airport, where I met him and drove him back to his house. The few weeks of separation had in many ways been a good thing for us, for we had both had time to ourselves for contemplation of our feelings. And that is why after three weeks of being apart from each other, and within the first ten minutes of being back in his Maiduguri house, we became engaged. Now at last, the station could really enjoy that much anticipated engagement party!

And finally, not having said anything to my parents about Rex, I wrote to them and dropped the bombshell, including the fact that we had decided to have our wedding in Maiduguri. Somehow it seemed right that way. Things moved at a cracking pace after that, or so it seemed to us.

Tom and Marjorie Letchworth, the Resident and his wife, had been out on tour when we got engaged, but as soon as they came back, they had us round one evening, and Marjorie asked, "Are you going to be married from the Residency? You'll be my fifth bride!" She was so kind to me – both of them were, keeping in touch, offering advice and insisting that when I had moved out of my house (which would be a few days before the wedding), I should stay in the Residency with them. "You will be able to come and go as you wish," they told me, "and we shall probably be out for some of the time so we won't be worrying you at all. It will be better than being in the Rest

House all that time." Thereafter, Tom, a tall, quiet and courteous man, and Marjorie, full of practical common sense, were superb. I couldn't have been looked after more lovingly if I had been their own daughter, and Marjorie – typically thoughtfully – wrote to our parents as well. We never forgot their kindness to us, which continued long after their retirement from overseas service in the form of correspondence from Marjorie.

The wife of a friend of ours, who had returned to the UK after a spell with him in Maiduguri, had managed to meet my mother, giving her all the up to date news of us. I asked our friend, who remained in Maiduguri to finish his tour of duty, if he would act for my father and 'give me away' at the wedding. None of our parents were able to travel to Nigeria, and we felt that this very slight link might make them feel a bit nearer to us on the day. Letters were exchanged between them and our friends, and I think our parents felt that they were involved a tiny bit in the proceedings as a result. We hoped so.

Women who held permanent appointments in Government Service, as I did then, were not allowed to remain in permanent posts if they married. They had to resign as from the day before the wedding and re-apply (if they wished to continue to work) for temporary employment as from the day after the ceremony. This was so that they could accompany their husbands when the latter were posted elsewhere, and also on leave. When going on leave, a married woman had to resign from her temporary employment each time, and re-apply for it on return, as well as for a new work permit each time. The terms of my present employment as a permanent serving officer meant that I had to give three months' notice if I resigned. The man Rex had replaced as PEO was due to return from leave at the beginning of September, and although we hoped that we might stay in Maiduguri, it was possible that he would come back to his old job and that Rex would be posted out. We wanted to be married by that time so that we would stay together wherever Rex might be sent to for a new posting. Three months from the day of our engagement brought us to the beginning of September as it happened, so we fixed our wedding day for 2nd September and I sent in my notice accordingly.

Suddenly there seemed an awful lot to be organised in a very short time. 'What shall you wear?' was the question on everyone's lips. What indeed? I would have been quite happy to be married in ordinary clothes, but Rex wanted it all 'proper', so the hunt was then on for a suitable dress pattern and material. Our faithful Butterick catalogue had a pattern, but Maiduguri had no wedding gown material in any of its canteens, nor in any of the local shops in the native town.

One of the air pilots undertook to get some samples from Lagos, while my mother, having recovered from the shock of my big announcement, sent several samples from home. It was one of hers that I finally selected.

148

Food for the reception? 'No problem at all,' said many of the wives and all the staff at the women's college and girls' school, 'we will all do something special for the day, don't worry about food, we will manage that between us.' It was amazing how much help was given and how many people ensured that September 2nd would indeed be a day Rex and I should never forget.

Louis, thoughtful as ever, said to me, "Now, girl, you'll need to do some shopping. I'm arranging for you to have a few days of local leave and you are to go to Jos for it. You'll be able to get what you need there." He booked me in at the Jos Catering Rest House and sent me off. I was going to have to get everything done in one day when in Jos, as the rest of the time allowed would be taken up with travelling. It would be a busy day. I did indeed get most of what I myself needed for the wedding, as well as (inevitably) shopping for many other people in station. I also got my car serviced for the first time ever, at the garage from which I had bought it. And I managed to buy a set of spare tyres for Rex, all of his others having had punctures in them more than once. I had to leave my car at the service garage for a whole day, and wondered how I was going to get to the canteens. I asked the service engineer if I could hire a car for the day, explaining why I was in Jos and telling him all the things I had to do. But he insisted that I borrow his car. "I shan't be going home until the end of the day," he told me, "so I won't need it at all until late. You don't need to bring it back until you come to collect yours." I thought it more than kind of him.

I managed, in addition to everything else, to find some very pretty material with which to make dresses for the little bridesmaids. "Bridesmaids?" I had asked Rex in surprise. Yes, he said, there must be bridesmaids. Our dental officer had two little daughters aged, I suppose, about four and six years old. Would they like to be bridesmaids? And would their parents allow them to? "Would they not!" said their Mum. "They've done nothing but play at weddings and bridesmaids recently as it happened. They'll be so excited now that their games are to happen for real." I wonder if they still remember, all these years later?

Would we have time for a honeymoon, we wondered, and if so, where could we go? We decided that the Southern Cameroons would be ideal. Rex wrote 'To Kaduna' asking if he could have some local leave – for some reason he didn't add that it would be for a honeymoon, so Kaduna therefore had no idea why he wanted local leave. It seemed, though, that for various reasons to do mainly with the timing of his return flight from the compassionate leave, he would not now be allowed to have any local leave for the remainder of his tour of duty, so there would be no honeymoon at all. But that didn't worry us really.

The next thing that happened was another letter to Rex from Kaduna to

149

say that Hugh Vernon Jackson (the man he had replaced) was returning from leave at the beginning of September and would be posted back to Maiduguri. Rex therefore was to proceed on September 2nd to a new station, Katsina. Rex wrote back by return to say that actually September 2nd was to be his wedding day. Oh, said Kaduna, we hadn't heard about that. Why didn't you say? In that case, you can have an extra 48 hours added to your travelling time before reporting in at the Katsina Training College. We actually spent much of the 48 hours in Kano, trying to sort out my income tax, which had become complicated in view of my change of status.

The next problem was that of where in Maiduguri we could be married. The little courthouse on the GRA, although used for Sunday services, was not licensed for weddings, so that was out. The Resident could marry us at his office in a civil ceremony, but we both wanted to be married in church if at all possible. We put out feelers and were thrilled when the local African Anglican congregation offered for us to be married in their little church, St John's Anglican Church, Maiduguri.

Next thing to arrange – who would marry us? Here we hit mega problems. The obvious person was the missionary clergyman from Molai, just a few miles up the road from Maiduguri. But no, unfortunately he was just about to go on leave and in fact was going on retirement so would not be returning. There was another mission out towards the Northern Cameroons, half a day's journey away. But again we drew a blank – the clergyman there was also to be on leave at the relevant time. Never mind, there were other mission stations – how about the one outside Jos, only a few hundred miles away? Well, sadly, no – the man there was going on leave as well, and didn't know if his replacement would have arrived by September 2nd. In any case, he couldn't commit his replacement to that sort of schedule. The Bishop of Northern Nigeria, Bishop Mort? Dare we approach him – would it be presumptuous of us to ask him? Well, nothing ventured, nothing gained, and we wrote to ask, and had a very nice letter back saying how pleased he would have been to come – but unfortunately he would be out of the country at the time.

The Archdeacon of Jos, perhaps? Very sorry, but his touring programme was already arranged and he would be elsewhere at the time, otherwise he would have come with pleasure. It looked as if we would have to have a civil wedding after all, conducted by the Resident in his capacity as Registrar. We both liked Tom Letchworth and knew he would conduct our wedding beautifully – but we both wished our marriage could have been in church. However, for the time being we had to leave it there.

Then one day, one of the charge nurses at the hospital, Mr Ndekwu, asked me, "Who will be marrying you, doctor?" I explained the situation and said how sad we felt about it. Mr Ndekwu was shocked. "But it is unthinkable that our doctor cannot be married in church.!" he exclaimed, "I will write to the Archdeacon myself!" (Mr Ndekwu was a devout churchman and a senior member of St John's congregation). And indeed he did write, showing me the letter before he posted it... 'Venerable Sir...' And lo and behold, Archdeacon Uzodike altered his schedule and drove to Maiduguri over waterlogged roads at the end of the rainy season, to give us a lovely marriage service. We never forgot his kindness.

A few days later, Mr Ndekwu, by now taking a very personal interest in my welfare, and making sure that everything else was going all right, took me discreetly on one side. "By the way, doctor," he said, "I do hope that Mr Abraham is paying the right price to your father for you. In my country here, a woman with a degree will cost as much as £200."

Everything now seemed to be organised and we relaxed. One of the nursing sisters, Kate Griffin, said to me that she would lend us a lace tablecloth for the wedding cake to stand on, and a knife with which to cut it that had only ever been used in her family to cut wedding cakes. Wedding cakes? My goodness, we hadn't thought about a cake! Should I try to make one? I was no good at baking at the best of times. Would anyone else be able to make one for us? We couldn't buy such things in Maiduguri. Mrs Letchworth, experienced in these matters (I was going to be her fifth bride after all), put her foot down. "No," she said firmly "It would never do to try to make one here – far too hot for that kind of baking. The cake wouldn't bake properly and the icing would never set. You must have a proper cake sent to you from Lagos. They put special preservatives in to stop them from going rancid and they do a special kind of icing that keeps hard too." So off went an order to the United Africa Company (UAC) in Lagos, who confirmed that they would supply a Huntley and Palmer wedding cake for the due date. I asked them to send it to Maiduguri no later than the penultimate plane, knowing that there could still be some rain and storms around then, and thinking that if the plane was cancelled because of the weather there would still be a last chance for the cake to arrive by the last plane.

My parents posted a pack of pretty invitation cards for us to send and, after correspondence with the Archdeacon, we settled on the hymns to be sung at the service. There was a small printing press in Maiduguri, amazingly, and we had some 'programmes' of the service printed all ready.

The material for my dress arrived from England, and our Health Sister, Anne Lamb, who was a wizard when it came to dressmaking, swept it out of my hands, grabbed the paper pattern and took it all to her house. "I shall make it up for you," she told me firmly, "because this one has got to fit. I'll

151

let you sew a bit of the hem." That, I felt, spoke volumes for my skill with anything other than a surgical needle!

Rex's mother packed and posted his best Sunday-go-to-meeting suit, which, though made for wear in Britain and not the tropics, he reckoned he could cope with for half a day in Maiduguri.

And finally, David Ani, who ran the little open-air cinema, said that he was shortly making a trip to Fort Lamy (now Ndjamena) in Chad, and would we like him to bring back a supply of good French wine for the reception? Indeed we would, and that was my first introduction to Vouvray wine, which of course I have enjoyed ever since.

Our work didn't stop just because we were in the throes of all these arrangements, and things continued as usual professionally for us both.

Louis made a final mad dash round the province to check all the bush dispensaries, before the rains hit really hard, while Rex also organised a three week tour up north as far as Lake Chad, to inspect schools there. During that time he had managed to have a trip on the lake in one of the local reed boats, which he was very pleased about. He found that tour to be very tiring and also very hot, and told me on his return that he was so hot and thirsty that he could almost see bottles of the local Star Beer dancing tantalisingly on the bonnet of his car as he drove! About this time too, our dentist went on tour to treat people in villages far out from Maiduguri. He had a special dental chair that could be dismantled and reassembled, and this was packed up together with instruments and other equipment ready for him to take with him. To my utter consternation, just as he was about to set off, he dashed into my office and pushed a small bundle into my hands. I opened it to find a set of tooth extraction forceps. "Those," he said, pointing to one side, "are for the upper jaw, and the others are for the lower jaw. It says on each which teeth they are for. Good luck" – and with that he was off. Upper jaw? Lower jaw? I'd never extracted a tooth in my life – how on earth...?

By the time he returned, I'd found out, though fortunately hadn't needed to take out more than a very few teeth. Well, we live and learn.

Some of our senior nurses were to be sent to the UK on various courses, courtesy, I think, of the British Council. I don't really know what training they'd had in Nigeria, except that it would probably not have been as comprehensive as that in England. Our matron took them all in hand for a few weeks to show them some of our English ways. There was so much that they needed to know. For instance, not one of them had ever eaten with a knife and fork – in Maiduguri people ate with fingers or spoons. Often one ate from a communal dish.

After he arrived in Britain, one of them wrote to Matron and told her that what he was doing was very hard work as compared with his job in Africa. Eventually he was transferred from his first base in the UK to do a course in tuberculosis at a hospital that was not far from Hull where my parents were, and they arranged for him to visit them. I was long gone from Maiduguri by the time he returned, so I never heard from him what he'd thought about the UK.

Everybody seemed to have seen Lake Chad but me, and ever since knowing that I was to come to Nigeria, I had wanted to visit the lake. It sounded very interesting. Not only were there reed islands on it where people lived, but it also had a special type of elephant there that had adapted to life in the watery and marshy surroundings. To borrow a phrase 'not many people knew that' but I found it fascinating. My first chance to see the lake came about now. Somebody else - perhaps the geologist, or maybe one of the engineers, I forget now, told me that he had to go up to the lake, and that as he was short of time he was doing the round trip in a chartered plane and would be there and back to Maiduguri in an afternoon. There would be a spare seat - would I like to go? Indeed I would. But - and there is always a but - Louis was already out on tour, and I was on my own at the hospital. If I went off for a few hours there would be no cover, and I could not let that happen. However, there was another doctor - the one who looked after Public Health, who was based out towards the Northern Cameroons. He came into Maiduguri every so often for a day or two, and I'd heard that he would be in town on the day in question. I wondered if he would be willing to cover for me. As luck had it, he didn't come to town that week after all, so very regretfully I had to decline the offer.

What a good thing I did, for the plane developed some problems and had to be grounded at a place called Geidam, way up to the north of the province. It was there for two or three days before repairs could be effected. It just so happened that Louis had arrived that same day at Geidam and was to stay there overnight before moving on to his next touring destination. I often wondered what his reaction would have been if I'd turned up and been stranded there when I was officially in charge of the General Hospital in Maiduguri. It wouldn't have been much good to say that I was only having a half day off. It's an ill wind...

An extraordinary case presented itself at the hospital one day. A horseman rode up to the office, followed by another man on foot. I noticed that the second man walked with a bit of a limp, but that was nothing untoward in a country of tropical ulcers that could cripple people, and also poliomyelitis, which was still rife, so that some had weakened muscles as a result. The rider leaned down from the saddle and asked me to look at the other man who he said had hurt his leg a week or so ago and it wasn't getting any better. The injured man pulled up his caftan to show me that one leg was heavily bandaged from hip to knee with all sorts of rags tied on with grasses. When we got these off I saw that there was neither wound nor deformity of any kind, and his muscles did not seem to be wasted particularly. I sent him for X-ray. To my astonishment, the film showed a healing fracture of the shaft of the femur. There was no displacement of the bone. I called Louis to see the film and to tell me that I wasn't seeing things that were not there. No, he confirmed that there was indeed a huge fracture. I was not surprised that it was still sore and that the patient didn't feel as if he was any better! The extraordinary thing was that the poor fellow had walked all the way from his village to Maiduguri for help – a distance of forty to fifty miles. The rider who had come with him as escort didn't appear to have offered him a lift either. The bandages had probably helped to hold everything in place and allowed healing to begin. We could hardly believe our eyes when we looked again at the X-ray. You just never knew what you would see next in our job.

I cannot now recall what we decided would be the best thing to do – but I'd guess that we probably kept him in hospital for a week or two so as to give a bit more time for the healing process before sending him back home. There was certainly no need by the time he arrived for anything else in the way of treatment. I think this shows how tough many people had to be, though, when they lived far from medical help. They simply accepted that things would and did happen to them and that they had to put up with what befell them. Either you recovered or you didn't. If you didn't, it was just too bad, but it was the will of Allah and had to be taken on board and one got on with it as best one could.

As the months went by and the rains really came down we had the usual run of cases of pneumonia. We also had the usual run of rainy season fractures.

Fractures? Why should there be more fractures in the rainy season? Well, because so many houses in the town, almost all really, were made of mud. The heavy rain softened some of the mud, so that bits of houses could collapse. If you were under a collapsing bit, then you were quite likely to have a bone broken – generally these were minor fractures, collar bones, forearms or ribs, but they all added to the general workload.

There was the usual constant stream of tropical ulcers. Our stock treatment then was daily dressings of Eusol (Edinburgh University Solution of Lime), which seemed to clear up the open sores and allow them to try to heal. But it took a long time. Although we also gave penicillin for some, the regular Eusol dressings seemed to be as good as anything, and often more effective than anything else anyway. I am sure that there are different treatments now and that Eusol would be thought to be very old fashioned. But it was all we had available for local application, and it worked more often than not. These ulcers were, when extensive, very crippling and many people's limbs, usually their legs, would be quite deformed by the chronic infection. For many, their bad legs which were often contracted and wasted, were their only means of livelihood, for they justified begging, and a good Moslem would always give if he possibly could, to a beggar. One saw many a beggar whose legs were permanently bent double at the knee, swinging himself or herself along the ground by holding a brick or a lump of wood in each hand which acted as a sort of shoe, I suppose. They would place the wood on the ground, and by taking their body weight on their hands, would swing their legs and body forward before sitting on the sand while they brought their hands forward to start the whole process again. Progress would be slow but not as slow as you might think. To use the wood meant that the palms of their hands didn't get as hard and rigid as the skin on the soles of those who walked on bare feet as most people did. The hands were needed for fine movements as well as for a means of 'walking', so the palmar skin had to remain supple.

Although many of the beggars were pitiably poor, most of them managed to keep themselves fed after a fashion. And I suppose many of them would have families who would give them food too. Many of the chronic ulcer sufferers were not keen to come to hospital, for they feared that if they were cured, or even half cured, their means of getting money would diminish and they felt that they couldn't afford for this to happen. However, in the end, the limbs could become so painful or so badly infected and toxic, that there were always a few in hospital who had to have a limb amputated. If we didn't do that for them, they would be in the end so debilitated and anaemic that they would die.

If we could, when amputating legs, we tried to do below-the-knee jobs. The reason for this was that there was no such thing as a prosthesis department anywhere, and for an artificial limb one had to depend upon local carpenters. The carpenters could make peg-legs quite well. What they did was to make the peg part and contrive a sort of kneeler at the top of it onto which the amputee would kneel with his knee bent rather than having a possibly ill fitting socket into which a bare stump would be inserted. Patients found the peg-leg plus kneeler far more comfortable and we found that they did not have problems with sore or raw stumps that way. As many of them lived far away from Maiduguri it was important that they went home able to manage without trouble from then on, for generally there would be no follow up. Many would end up by not using the artificial 'leg' at all, but would contrive a sort of crutch for themselves and manage with that alone. The other aspect of this system was also that of cost. Prostheses as we think of them would have been beyond any affordability then. I wonder if things have changed in the last forty or so years.

It was interesting to see how, very frequently, a patient's overall condition improved once a badly infected limb was off and the toxic focus had gone. It was also interesting to realise how people in general seemed to adapt to being anaemic. They got accustomed, presumably, to being below par and functioned at that level, apparently doing all their normal tasks as usual. Yet if they attended the clinic for any reason, and a blood count was ordered by the doctor, it was found that many needed treatment to correct their blood picture. We didn't at that time have facilities for blood transfusion in Maiduguri, and in any case, families were never keen on the idea of giving blood. Once in desperation I did ask family members if they would be willing to give blood for a relative, if we could get her and them to somewhere like Kano or Lagos, where I felt that transfusion would be possible, but I got a very indifferent response. Clearly the idea was not welcome. In any case, what other infections might have been transferred in given blood? It was not a simple thing to think about by any means. Well, the question didn't really arise as we had neither the lab potential nor the ward skills available, to say nothing of proper storage facilities.

I often thought it surprising how much we did achieve on the whole. There was so little general knowledge about health and hygiene, though the people were very cleanly inclined and swept and tidied their compounds regularly, and if water was easily available, washed their clothes as often as they could. Small children were made to stand in big enamel bowls while their mothers sluiced them with water and kept them as clean as they could. But often water was too precious to 'waste' by using it for washing. It had to be conserved for drinking and cooking purposes. In many villages, water was only obtainable from wells, and the women had to spend a lot of time collecting what they needed for the day. Sometimes there were water carriers who filled used kerosene cans with water and carried it round to households where they would sell it. But poor people couldn't afford to buy so had to carry their own. It seemed extraordinary how scarce water could be when one realised that there was plenty underground. It was tapped from deep artesian wells, and there were standpipes in the town which were used, but not so many in or near villages.

In the senior service houses we had a proper water supply on tap, but even so, the water was very often cut off during the day and came on again at about teatime. Our practice at home was to get all the laundry done early and then fill the bath so that we had water available during the day for all purposes. Then after about 4 p.m., we could once again use the taps and all was well.

At one time, some of the senior students from the Bornu Teacher

Training College were sent out to nearby villages for teaching practice. We were surprised to see them coming back to college most evenings, having borrowed bicycles for the journeys. When we asked why they kept coming back, sometimes distances of twenty miles or so, they told us it was to get water. In the villages, they said, they often had to buy water from the local carriers, and as students, found the cost to be more than they could afford. It was cheaper by far to hire bicycles and return to Maiduguri after the day's work was done, in order to get water to carry back. This is something we don't think about in the UK. How lucky we are.

Chapter 19

We came to the last week in August. I started to go to the airport to meet the last planes in case our wedding cake arrived early, but nothing came. The penultimate plane, as I had feared, was indeed cancelled because of tropical storms. Apprehensively Rex and I drove down to the airport to meet the very last plane in. It was the day before our wedding. The plane landed, the passengers disembarked and their luggage was off loaded, but there was nothing for me. I dashed into the air traffic controller's office. No, nothing had arrived - sorry. The pilot returned to his aeroplane and took off for Yola, his next stop. Disbelievingly I watched the aircraft soar into the sky and quickly become no more than a dot that soon disappeared. Other people got into their cars and drove away.

I was bitterly disappointed, and probably very frustrated as well - I had tried so hard to have everything perfect. Rex made reassuring noises - it was only a cake, he said, and not the end of the world. Then suddenly, as we were turning disconsolately back to the car, I saw a small wooden crate far out - almost on the runway. I ran across the tarmac and looked at it. No label, no address, nothing. It was totally anonymous. Just as I was about to go back to the car, I noticed some faint pencilling at the bottom of one side of the crate. I bent down. The letters were upside down. Craning my neck I managed to make out the words 'two tier'.

"It's it!" I yelled, "What else but a wedding cake would have two tiers!"

And despite the protestations of the air traffic controller, we grabbed it and bore it off to the Residency where by that time I was living. And sure enough, it was the cake - all packed in tin boxes within wooden boxes, separated by wads of packing and padding.

"There won't be time to unpack it and set it up anew tomorrow," said Mrs Letchworth, "But how will we stop the ants getting at it overnight if we set it up this evening? The fridge isn't big enough and anyway it will be being filled up with food for tomorrow."

After a few minutes of thinking: "I know," she said, "There is another spare bathroom upstairs. We'll set it up and stand it in the bath full of water. I have a tall metal stand somewhere that we can use."

And that is what we did. I have a photograph of it on the metal stand in the bath, flanked by the washbasin, hot water geyser and loo, where it remained all night. And not one ant found it.

The wedding day went off beautifully. I started by seeing a last patient or two, and then called round at various houses to collect the food that different friends had prepared. It was soon time to get ready. Rex and I both felt it to be wonderfully appropriate having met and become engaged in Africa, now to be married by an African priest in an African church, surrounded by all our friends, among whom were Africans, both Moslem and Christian, as well as expatriates. And it didn't rain for twenty four hours.

How hard both Tom and Marjorie Letchworth worked to make things go well for us! Marjorie, I knew, had been up at the crack of dawn on the great day to look for flowers in the Residency grounds so that she could make the bouquet and sprays. It being the back end of the rainy season, there were still some flowers available, and I was enchanted to be given a lovely bouquet of pink and white striped lilies that grew wild in the bush, dianthus, trailing coralita, and little pink rambler roses.

The Resident had lent me his car together with a Native Authority police driver to take me to the church, where the Federal Police were on duty to organise the parking of all the guest's vehicles. We found that the local congregation had painted up the inside of the church for us, and had widened the drive so that it could take the number of cars anticipated. We hadn't expected anything like that and were very touched. We had been given another lovely surprise as well. Ray Underwood, who wrote the foreword to this book, had just returned from leave. He had brought back with him the first tape recorder any of us had seen - reel to reel jobs they were then – and he offered to tape the service for us on one of his precious spare reels as a wedding gift. However, before he could do so, he needed an electricity supply. The church had none. The local manager of the ECN (Electricity Corporation of Nigeria) was told about the problem, and said that if the church congregation would allow it, he would bore a hole in the church wall and run a temporary cable through for the occasion. And this is what happened, so we had a lovely memento of the whole occasion, which was great for us, but which also meant that we could let our families hear it all when we went home on leave. Two other friends followed us round with cine-cameras as well, so in addition to snapshots we had the films to show afterwards as well. The little church had no organ for music, but another friend - how gallant she was! - volunteered to play the music for the service on a small harmonium worked by foot pedals - no mean task because it was so hot. And play she did - music before our arrival, music for the hymns, music to keep everyone going while we were in the vestry signing the register, and music for us to walk back through the church to the waiting car when all the ceremony was over. On the tape recording of it all, there are moments when you can hear her pedalling away as she played, and I always think when

I hear it how exhausted she must have been afterwards.

Our guests included people from several nationalities – English, French, Lebanese, and Africans among others. We were specially pleased to see that our Moslem African friends came into the church and took part in the service. We were also pleased to see the proprietor and his wife from a tiny shop just next to the hospital where, at mid morning break, Rex (whose office was just across the road from the hospital) and I would go to buy cans of cool drinks if we didn't feel like imbibing the hot coffee which was always served in Matron's office at that time.

Just before we returned to the Residency for the reception, Rex and I were driven to the hospital where the staff, who could not come to the church, had asked to see us. We stood outside the office and everyone queued up to shake our hands and wish us well – and I suppose to see what we looked like in our finery.

It was a very happy occasion for us. Rex didn't know everyone as I did, but even I didn't recognise the last man in the line of people waiting. When he came along, my new husband put out his hand and the man held out his – but he was holding an envelope. Then "Sorry, Sir," he said, and handed over the envelope. It was Rex's final electricity bill, his house just having been closed down. We all laughed. But he shook hands with us like everyone else and wished us well.

Later, when Mrs Letchworth produced all the cablegrams and telegrams that had arrived for us, there was amongst them one from the local postmaster who had been receiving them and sending them up to the Residency:

'Mr Mrs Abraham Residency Maiduguri
Happy Days and Best Wishes.
Mephe Postoffice.'

The reception over, we set out in our two cars en route for Katsina. We had worried a bit about the journey, it still being the rainy season so that there was always the possibility of being held at the barriers along the road. However, another friend, one of the assistant superintendents of the Nigerian Police, had passed there a few days previously, and had told the gatekeepers that we were to be allowed through, explaining why. The road was pretty waterlogged in places and we found ourselves driving through quite deep water. But every barrier was opened for us and we were waved through with greetings of "Aure! Aure!" which meant "Wedding! Wedding!" It was all great fun. On the way we also met Hugh Vernon Jackson, who, his leave finished, was now returning to Maiduguri to take over his old job. We stopped to exchange news. Hugh produced an unopened bottle of rather good whisky from his loads, and we had flasks of coffee with us. We combined the two and had another little party on the roadside while Rex gave a verbal handing-over to supplement the notes he had left for Hugh in the PEO's office.

We were taking Ali our cook and Momso, our small boy in the cars with us, as well as our menagerie of animals. Rex was a cat lover and had two cats, Flora and Fauna, for which we had a huge box made. They were in the box in the back of my estate car, while my dog rode in Rex's car on Ali's knee at the front. The little dog loved being in the car and was always as good as gold when travelling. At prearranged intervals we stopped on the road for a breather. Accordingly, Rex pulled in to the bush at the side of the road and waited for me to catch up. I stopped several yards behind his car and got out. Seeing that my dog had been let out and was dashing delightedly all over the place, smelling new smells and seeing new things, I called him. He stopped, looked around, and then came galloping to me, wagging his tail and showing great excitement before jumping up to me and greeting me in his doggy way.

Coming along on the other side of the road was an old man, driving a few cows in front of him. He saw all this happening and watched closely. Then he crossed over and spoke to Ali for a few minutes. Ali came to us, chuckling. "This man says he has never before seen a dog that knew its name," he told us, "and he says will Madam sell it to him for one of his cows." Well, I kept my dog and he kept his cow as you will realise. But I couldn't help smiling to myself at the thought of trying to stuff a cow into the car and taking it to Katsina with us.

All driving done but for the last lap of our transfer to Katsina, we stopped for our extra forty eight hours at the Central Hotel in Kano. Rex had been stationed in Kano some years before, and knew several people there, so we were well entertained in the evenings and had a most enjoyable time. Then we drove the last one hundred miles to our new home. Rex was to work at the Katsina Men's Training College, which was quite a prestigious place from all I could gather. The students there always prided themselves on their spoken English – 'Katsina English' as it was then known. The college buildings were fairly new and everything was quite impressive.

Rex, in addition to his lecturing duties was made deputy Principal and also college bursar, which meant a lot of bookwork and financial tasks. It made for an interesting job overall, albeit a busy one. Busy for both of us in fact, for we were often asked to put up VIP visitors – Chief Inspectors of schools, colleges and others of similar rank. On two or three occasions when the Principal had to be away for a short time, Rex had to take on his duties. At such times if there were any special events at the college such as inter-collegiate sports, we had to organise evening parties for fifty or more people.

It was always easy to accommodate them because we could generally hold the party out in the compound, knowing that there would be no rain or wind for nine months of the year. There was no street lighting of course, so we would light up the driveway like a small flare path, with candles standing in empty tins which would be plunged into the sand (baked bean tins were always useful). We knew that nothing would blow the candles out. Then we would have the main party as near to the house as we could so that light from the windows would stream out, and we would have Tilley lamps set down here and there outside as well. If we were lucky the electricity manager would fix up an outside light for the evening.

Our house was one of three that were not on the GRA but instead were on the edge of the town within walking distance of both our places of work. Two of these, ours and one in the next compound were allocated to education officers at the college, while the third nearby was occupied by the headmaster of the Boys' Secondary School. His wife was a real gardening expert who had, with the help of a garden boy, transformed her sandy compound into a riot of colour with flowers and shrubs of all kinds. She managed to keep it looking constantly fresh and luxuriant because she had the garden boy busy watering it for a great deal of the time. It was an experience to see what could be done if you had the skill to visualise it and the time to attend to it.

The GRA, where the senior service officers were quartered in Katsina, was a mile or two out of the town. There was just one small canteen there from which we could get our household supplies. With Kano being so near (only one hundred miles away!) people tended to wait until they could spare a day to go there and do a bulk buy. The canteens were very good in Kano and you could find all sorts of little luxuries if you had time to look for them.

To reach our house we had to turn off the main roadway to the little mud walled town of Katsina, and up a road signposted 'To the Lunatic Asylum'. Would that be our house, we wondered. There were times when it might well have been, we thought as time went on, but actually the Lunatic Asylum was a little way beyond our house although on the same road. I was asked to take over the supervision of the patients there in addition to my regular hospital work. Poor souls, there was not much we could do for them really. Usually I had found that families looked after their own who were slightly deranged, although other 'mad' people would be found wandering about, perhaps stripped naked, perhaps wearing raggedy clothes, and almost all with their hair grown long and unkempt. They seemed to get food from anyone who would give, and were quite harmless generally. But there were those who could be violent, or who could not look after themselves at all and who were brought to the hospital for help. In Katsina such people were then housed in the 'Asylum' to be cared for by several attendants there. Each patient had a small room in which they spent most and sometimes all of their time. Some were allowed out into the compound, which was surrounded by a wall so that they could not get out into any public areas, and they would sit in a patch of shade thinking goodness knows what kind of thoughts. However there were others who could not be let out of their rooms at all because they were just so dangerous to other people. When I went round the first time, I went into most of the rooms to try to greet the patients and make some attempt to assess them. But the attendants refused to unlock the door of one man's room. They said, "You must not try to go in there, doctor. The last time a stranger went in, he was grabbed, and swung round the room against the walls and badly injured."

All we had that could be used for any treatment, and that was sedation only, was a new drug, Largactil. We had no psychiatric help at all, so it was really beyond any of us to make proper diagnoses and one just had to do the best one could to keep these poor individuals clean, quiet and fed. The attendants were really very good on the whole. We had no facilities for occupational therapy, which might have been very helpful. I felt particularly helpless in regard to the patients, not having any psychiatric experience myself, and felt that the most I could do for them was to make sure they were well looked after and properly cared for. I was always conscious of the fact that they needed much more than any of us could give them.

Some years later, when we were back in Maiduguri I heard that there was a specialist psychiatrist in Zaria. Katsina was accessible for anyone living in Zaria who had a car. I wondered if he or she ever went to Katsina to 'my' Lunatic Asylum.

I had been re-employed on a 'temporary' basis, and a fortnight after our arrival in station I started work at the Katsina General Hospital. It was a bit larger than that in Maiduguri, and its compound was more extensive too. I particularly liked the theatre block, the operating theatre itself being larger and much lighter and cooler than had been the case in Maiduguri. The two senior nurses there were both very capable men. One of them, Mallam Manda, acted as theatre sister and was first assistant to whichever doctor was operating if there was no other medical officer to assist. Mallam Manda did his job extremely well – and I may say that the instruments were always properly boiled up. His colleague, whose name to my shame I cannot now recall, would give the anaesthetics unless there was a spare doctor to do the 'dopes'. He gave an excellent anaesthetic, and I never really worried about patients under his care, although needless to say I and the other MOs always kept a good eye on what was going on at the head end of the patient. Between them, these two nurses made a very good team.

My habit in Katsina was to start my regular theatre list at 10 a.m., straight after the breakfast break. I would poke my nose round the theatre door just before dashing home for breakfast to say, "I'll be back to start at ten sharp don't forget." But they were never ready then – clocks didn't seem to matter much in Africa. I was always thinking however of the myriad jobs I would still have to tackle after my theatre list.

One day, however, when I returned, I saw that they were in theatre, all scrubbed up and gowned. The patient was already on the table, towelled up and the skin already painted up with iodine. As I walked in, I saw that the anaesthetist nurse had the lint-covered mask over the patient's face and the bottle of chloroform poised ready for the first drop to fall on it. The patient rolled his eyes round above the mask to look at me – did I detect a glint of amusement there? The others were chuckling. Mallam Manda selected a scalpel and held it out to me.

The anaesthetist dropped the first drop of chloroform onto the mask, pointedly looked at his watch and in a solemn tone of voice pronounced, "Ten sharp – England time!" I knew that I had really been accepted if they felt that they could pull my leg.

The Emir of Katsina was a much younger man than the Shehu of Bornu. Protocol demanded that in addition to going to sign the Resident's book in Katsina, I also had to be formally presented to the Emir. Dr Furness, the medical officer in charge, took me to the Emir's palace, where we were conducted to his Reception Chamber. This was a long high room, very light and airy. At the far end sat the Emir on a throne-like chair, with many attendants sitting on the floor round him. We were signalled to stop just as we'd got into the room. Then our escort approached the Emir, prostrating himself on the floor as he did so. He very respectfully announced us.

The Emir, speaking in Hausa, asked Dr Furness to introduce me. We were not bidden to approach the Emir ourselves. The Emir turned to me and expressed his wish, again in Hausa, that I would be happy in Katsina. I thanked him. Then we were dismissed.

As we were about to leave, another attendant came to me. "The Emir wants you to be taken to his wives' compound to meet his wives. Come with me," he said. The wives' compound was a jolly place, almost like a village. There were many small buildings there. Some were the various domains of each wife and her children, while others were their kitchens (each wife would have her own kitchen) and others would be latrines, storerooms and so on. I was invited into the 'house' of the senior wife. The walls inside were covered with brightly covered enamel plates – signifying her own personal wealth, I was told. Some of the women were sitting out in the compound, spinning yarn, manipulating their distaffs and other bits of equipment with hands and toes alike. It looked difficult to me but I imagine the process fell into the category of 'It's really very easy once you know how.'

The most any of them could say in English was 'Good morning' or 'How are you?', but with that and my elementary Hausa we managed to spend a little time on a friendly basis. It seemed that I was the first female doctor there had been in Katsina and apparently the Emir was very pleased about this because I, unlike the male doctors, could (and would) be asked to visit the compound if any of the wives or children were ill. I was indeed called in from time to time – luckily never for much more than aspirin and anti-malarials would sort out. Often I thought that they just wanted a visitor – and I suppose for them I would be quite an exotic visitor just as in those days one of them if transported to the UK would be seen as exotic in her turn. Anyway we all seemed to enjoy my visits there. It was there too that I discovered the Emir was able to speak perfectly good English, for he was sometimes about there when I went.

Alhaji Usman Nagogo, the Emir, was a brilliant polo player. Every week there would be polo – generally the Emir's team versus the Europeans. Watching the Emir play, if it isn't too purple a phrase, was like seeing poetry on horseback – he really did seem to be one with his animal. As indeed, did his second in command, an older man with a grizzled beard, lean and athletic, who also flew up and down the field on his horse as if possessed. The Katsina team had, in fact, won the Nigeria Polo Association Georgian Cup in 1958, that very year, so everyone was pretty chuffed about it. Polo days were quite a social event in Katsina – we would all go to the field to watch, Africans and Europeans alike, as indeed we would all go to watch the Katsina races which, like those in Maiduguri, were great fun. Even Rex, who disliked horses and who had never ridden anything more than a seaside donkey, would come with me, threatening that he was only banking up polo and race days against the football matches he planned to take me to in England (I hate football!).

The nurse in charge of the female outpatients department was a jolly young Hausa woman with a great sense of humour. We were amused, she and I, when I was told that her name was Kati, upon which I was able to tell her that back in the UK, some of my friends would call me Katy. She was vivacious, hard working, and luckily for me, a great mimic. Although I spoke enough Hausa to cope with a clinic – well, mostly anyway – Kati often spoke so quickly and also often used several alternative words for syndromes so that I didn't always pick up what she'd said. She would then resort to mime, very successfully I may say and often much to my amusement. One day she told me that the next patient had 'gudu'. This was a new one on me. "Gudu?" "Yes," said Kati, and seeing that I still didn't understand, she acted out somebody suffering from acute and urgent diarrhoea (which I had been taught was '*zau*'). No doubt then about what she was trying to tell me. If I'd thought, I would have guessed because '*gudu*' means 'to run'.

The work was no different from that in Maiduguri. Serious cases were often things that were only mentioned in English textbooks of the day as having happened once upon a time but not really any more. Many of ours would be just these rarities, such as midwifery cases coming in from bush villages – babies with impossible presentations, babies half born and dead by the time they arrived at the hospital, women with septicaemia because of incomplete delivery of the placenta, and so on. The midwifery forceps that I had been given along with other bits of equipment when I left Beverley were to come into use more than once.

We had the usual admissions of people with fractured limbs who had been splinted (often very beautifully) by 'native doctors' in their villages. Sadly, however, the bandages would have been put on so tightly that the circulation was occluded and the limbs became gangrenous and had to be amputated. This was always a sad thing to see because the 'native doctors' so clearly had the right ideas and reduced the fractures very well before binding them up in splints. Unfortunately they did not have sufficient knowledge to go along with their ideas and instincts. How wonderful it would have been to be able give them some simple training. But there was never time to think about that sort of thing.

Here I will interpolate a short account of three amputations that I had to do during my years in Nigeria – all in youngsters, and all things that should never have been allowed to happen.

The first case was that of a tiny baby only a few weeks old. It was brought to the hospital with the story that it had 'crawled into the fire and got burnt.' On further questioning, I found that because it was Harmattan and the nights were cold, the family had taken to sleeping round a communal fire for warmth. This new little baby had been with its mother. When she woke in the morning, the baby was lying very close to the embers, and its right arm was charred – or rather, what was left of its arm was charred because the soft tissue of the lower and part of the upper arm had gone altogether, leaving burnt bone ends to be dealt with. I had to take the child into theatre and 'tidy' up what remained, which effectively meant an amputation of part of the remaining bit of the arm. The baby healed up well, but what a tragedy for it to start out on its life with a handicap that it should never have sustained.

The next instance was that of a young healthy lad of about twelve years old, who had broken his leg some days earlier. The local 'doctor' in his village had actually set the fracture extremely well and on X-ray the bones were seen to be in good alignment. The leg had been bound up with some sort of bandages over excellent makeshift splinting that had been made by using long straight thin branches from some bush or tree. So far so good, and the local medicine man had done a great job there. However, unfortunately he had fastened the binding far too tightly, no doubt hoping that firm bandaging would keep the leg straight. The result was that the limb became gangrenous and by the time the lad was brought to us there was no question of saving it. In order to save his life, I had to take his leg off. Another tragedy that should never have happened – and an event which would affect that boy's life from then on.

The third case in this series was that of a young girl, perhaps sixteen or so years old. She was brought to us in a moribund state, with a leg almost destroyed by a huge tropical ulcer, badly infected and gangrenous. I didn't rate much for her chances of survival actually, for she was so far gone that I thought she might not even survive the rest of that day. However, we started to treat her as best we could and I felt that if she survived the next few hours, I would risk taking her into theatre. To my astonishment, when I went later on to see how things were, she was sitting up in bed, fully alert and clearly in an enormously improved condition. I couldn't understand how this had happened even with the help of dressings and massive antibiotics. What had happened was that the affected leg had suddenly dropped off. Without that toxic focus, her body had gone into recovery mode and she was able to battle the debilitation that it had caused her. Yes, I had to take her into theatre, again to do a tidying up job, but she was another young person who recovered and went home. However, had she been brought to us for help when her ulcer had first started, she would very likely have gone into the rest of her life with two sound legs. What a lot needed to be done in Northern Nigeria at that time before we could help people as much as we wanted to.

The unexpected continued to happen, whether it was to do with patients or procedures. One day I had arranged a longish operating list. When I arrived at the theatre ready to start (no doubt at ten sharp!), it was to be told that the hospital ambulance, which normally transported our patients from ward to theatre and back again afterwards, had broken down and could not be used. So I had to fold down the back seats of my estate car, drive to the wards, load a patient into it, drive back across the compound to the theatre block, offload the patient, dash inside and scrub up, operate, then discard my gown and rubber apron before loading the unconscious person into the back of the car again and going back to the ward. This was repeated for every patient that morning. I thought we would never finish. It was a long hot day.

I have not yet said what provision there was for treating senior service personnel in Katsina. We had no nursing home as in Maiduguri, and anything serious or which needed inpatient treatment had to go to Kano. After all, Kano was only a hundred miles away, or two and a half hours in the car as you bumped over the potholed tarmac. In Nigeria that seemed to be no distance at all. We had a small room separate from the wards where we would see any Senior Service officers who came down for advice, or we would visit them at home on the GRA. Occasionally, if somebody was not too ill, I 'admitted' them to our spare room at home, where I could look after them myself. Our house was only about five minutes from the hospital, so that I could be home very quickly if needed.

Katsina itself was a walled town, the walls being made of mud, with several gateways in them. A lot of the mud was crumbling, and from time to time I would see men doing a repair job. One would be on top of and astride the wall, while others below would be moulding wet mud into huge balls, which they would throw up one at a time to the man aloft. He would then fit it onto the top of the wall and beat it into position where it would dry and harden in the sun. It was a time consuming job and a very hot tiring one, I should think. Within the walls Katsina was always busy. There was a thriving little market, full of people buying, selling, talking, walking, everyone active. Not far from the market were the 'dye-pits'. These were deep holes in the ground, full of dark liquid into which lengths of cloth were plunged to be dyed a dark purple colour. Outside the walls were the polo ground and the race course.

One of the gateways through the thick mud wall into town was known as the 'Lugard Gate' and outside there was a small plinth with a plaque on it saying that it was the place where Lord Lugard first entered Katsina. Lugard must have been quite a chap from what I have read and heard. He it was who stopped many of the local chiefs from having slaves, and as I understand it, many of the ordinary people were more than thankful as a result.

A few events stand out in my mind from my Katsina days. One was of the time when we received an invitation to a cocktail party at the Emir's Chamber. The Emir's Chamber was in fact a very nice modern bungalow, which was within his main compound. I had the impression that it was probably only for the use of visitors and not lived in by the Emir himself, though I stand to be corrected on that one. All the departmental heads and some others had been invited and the assembly was a mix of expatriates and Africans alike. On arrival we were welcomed in by his aide-de-camp, a Hausa man in the usual flowing robes, who took us on a conducted tour all round the house so that we might see how well it was fitted up. No expense had been spared – the furniture was good quality, the carpets were deep and soft. We were taken to see the bedrooms, and the softness of the beds was demonstrated to us by our guide who sat and bounced up and down on them, just to show. We were taken into the kitchens and cupboards were thrown open so that we could admire the beautiful chinaware that was displayed on the shelves

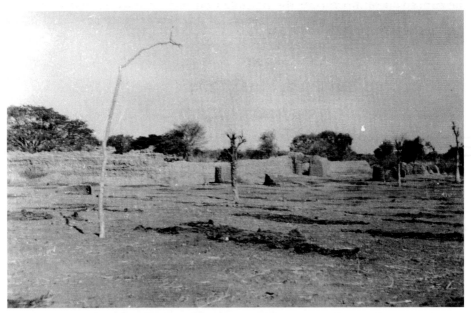

Gorgoram, a dying town - buildings crumbling, population leaving, desert taking over. March 1958.

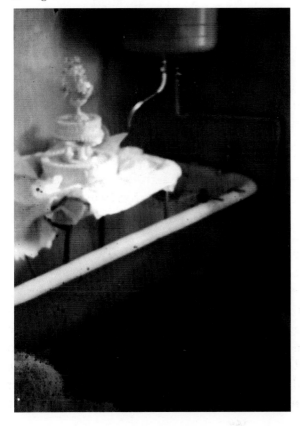

September 1st 1958.
The wedding cake stood in its glory overnight in a bath full of water in order to escape marauding ants.

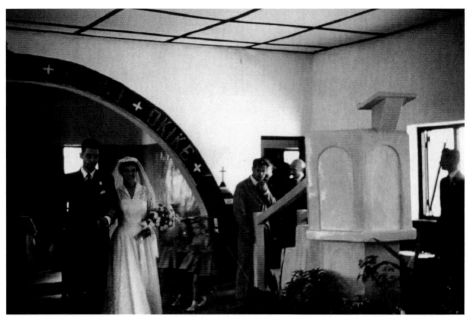

September 2nd 1958. My wedding to Rex in St John's Church, Maiduguri. 'Chuku Okike' means 'God the Creator'. To the left of the pulpit, in a light suit, is Ray Underwood, who wrote the foreword to this book.

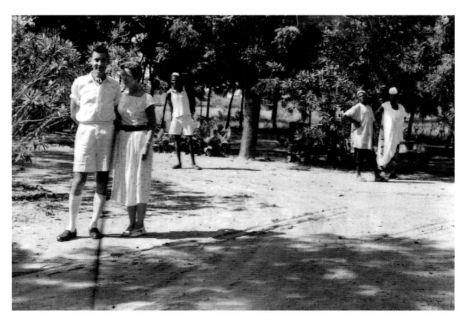

At Potiskum Rest House, the day after our wedding.

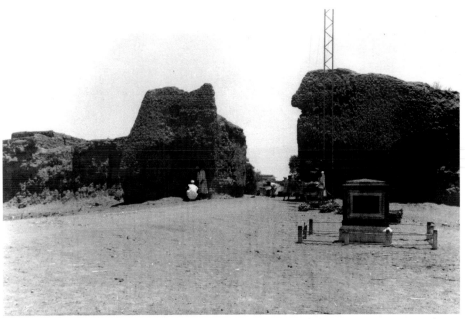

Lugard Gate and memorial, Katsina. It was through this gate that Lord Lugard entered Katsina in 1903.

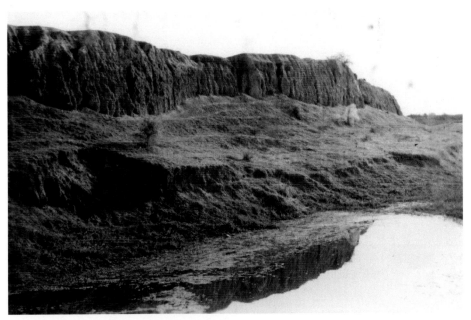

The old mud built walls of Katsina.

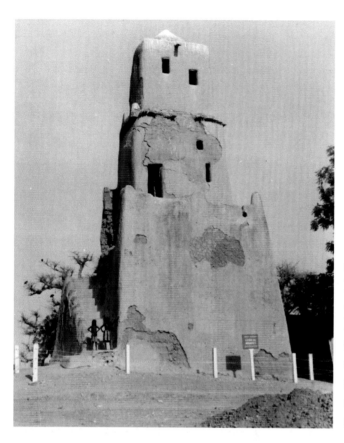

Gobarau Minaret, Katsina, hundreds of years old. It was not permitted to go up to the top as it was no longer safe to do so. I was able to get half way up . . .

. . . and took the photograph below.
The minaret overlooked a mud built primary school (foreground), with a general view of Katsina beyond.

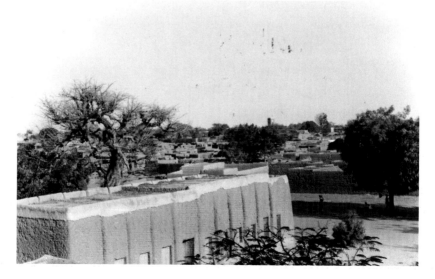

inside. It really was a dream house.

It was all rather fun to be there. Being a Moslem affair, there were no alcoholic drinks, and we were given either squash or Krola, which was the Nigerian equivalent of Coca-Cola. The evening was conducted with formality. The Emir and Native Authority officers circulated and spoke to everyone there, and eventually, as with similar occasions at the Residency, a discreet signal was put out to indicate that the evening was at an end.

Another exciting time was when we heard that there was to be a durbar at Daura, a small town about fifty miles away. The event, in either late 1958 or early 1959, was to be on one of the public holidays so that we knew we could be free to go. Rex and I, together with a friend, set off early in the morning before breakfast, and arrived just as things were almost ready to start. We were lucky in that we found ourselves guided to a place almost next to the Emir of Daura himself, therefore we had an ideal viewpoint. We were seated on a small dais at the bottom of a small tower-like edifice, and looking round, I noticed that there were some stairs up to the roof of it. Perhaps it was really a minaret. Anyway, while things happened, I managed to creep up to the top from where I could see the entire durbar and take some photographs and cine-film of the proceedings, so I was very pleased about that.

The usual display of horsemanship took place – line upon line of galloping horses coming towards the Emir from the far end of the local Dandal Way, with all the district heads in their finest robes. There were jesters and entertainers too – some stilt walkers being among them – in fact they were walking on some of the longest, highest stilts I had ever seen. Very impressive they were. Afterwards we were taken on a small tour of Daura, and especially to see what we were told was a sacred well there – sacred I seem to remember, to snakes. Eventually, when we had seen everything we could, we drove back to Katsina – and our breakfast. It had been a good morning.

While we were in Katsina, there was an eclipse of the sun – on September 30th 1959. This was an exciting thing to happen, and we all – the expatriate community that is – looked forward tremendously to seeing this not very frequent phenomenon. I was sorry not to be in Maiduguri where the eclipse would be total, but nonetheless we did pretty well in Katsina where it was a 95% eclipse. Our houseboys too had heard about it, and were also quite excited. I was surprised when, during the previous few days, Momso, our young 'small boy' who had never seemed to get worked up about anything, produced a fragment of broken glass which he had smoked, all ready to look through it at the sun on the appointed day. He, Ali and Audu our steward were all set to come into the compound and take turns with the smoked glass as the eclipse proceeded.

The Resident, Oliver Hunt, realised that much of the local populace might not understand the movements of celestial bodies, and some might be alarmed. Eclipses of the sun didn't happen so often that everyone would know about them or have seen one. So he sent a message to the Katsina Training College asking if the students could be instructed to go into the town and explain to the local people what was going to happen, why it would happen, and that it would pass, leaving everything as normal once more. The students happily did this. In spite of the care and thoughtfulness of the Resident and the work done by the students, there were still people in the town who were afraid. One man, we heard, had been so sure that if the sun blacked out it would be the end of the world, that he went so far as to sell up his house and all his possessions so that at least he would have the money when everything else ended. And we discovered that because the message delivered to the townspeople by our students had come from the Resident, many other people decided that the British, in fact, had something to do with the coming eclipse – otherwise how would they have known about it?

It happened at about 12 noon on the day, when the sun was at its highest and hottest. Gradually the light altered and the sky became almost copper coloured, I recall. I had managed to get hold of some old used X-ray film, and although we know nowadays that looking through smoked glass or film can still be harmful, we didn't know then, and so we all peered happily through what we had managed to find. At the peak of the eclipse, I could just see a tiny sliver of a crescent where the sun should be, but even that was enough to produce a lot of light, and the world was by no means obscured. Nevertheless, there was a very strange feeling everywhere. Somehow the atmosphere seemed to be very still and there was not a sound to he heard anywhere except that of our own voices. I remember too, thinking to myself 'I can feel something like a great pulsation in the air, what can that be?' Of course I never knew whether that was just me imagining things or if there was indeed some weird alteration in the atmosphere. Eventually, the sun gradually reappeared so that we could no longer look at it, and the day went on as usual. I often wondered what the man thought who had sold up his goods and chattels – and his house – when within an hour or two everything was just as it had always been. Was he able to buy things back?

Another subject that comes into my mind is that of the various ways in which people travelled when they were in need of hospital attention. The Mammy Wagons often had planks of wood fitted across them at the back, to act as benches so that they could carry passengers instead of goods. For cheapness, therefore, they were used by most people as the main means of mechanical transport. Railways were few and far between, and only went between the bigger towns. Only rich men could afford cars or air travel. Most of the ordinary folk got around on their own two feet, or by donkey or on horseback, if they owned a horse. Many undertook enormous journeys in order to get to a hospital. Some lines from one of my letters at the time explain:

'21.10.1958

I have a patient in now, with a dislocated neck...this woman came from bush and had been on the go for 24 hours before she got here, and I think she may be permanently paralysed in three limbs'

[I compared this case with an almost identical one I'd had in England, but where the patient was in the hospital within half an hour of the accident, and who was lucky enough to recover totally after treatment was started very quickly.]

The letter continued:

'Another patient has just arrived who has travelled for a whole day (yesterday) on horseback to get here. They come enormous distances to hospital from bush. We had an old man came to see me in Maiduguri who had travelled by donkey for five days and had then walked for two more days more before he got there.'

Travel itself, whether to hospital or elsewhere, was not without risk. Imagine the chaos when a Mammy wagon skidded in the sand, or turned over and flung everyone out. The injured from one such accident were brought to us just as I had arrived to do my evening round of the hospital. About twenty people injured in all sorts of ways were decanted onto the floor outside the operating theatre. I was the only doctor in station at the time. 'Triage' wasn't a word that we used then, we just sorted out the worst from the least worst cases and treated accordingly.

Among others there were five or six fractured femurs, all, I remember, in young men. I don't think we even had enough Thomas' splints in the hospital to cope with them all, and a bit of make do and mend had to be organised. One, sadly, was so badly smashed up with soft tissue injuries as well as the fracture that his leg had to come off. There was no way we could have got him to Kano – our ambulance was out of action, and he was in no state to be transported. He was resuscitated as well as was possible while I dealt with the rest of the injured. I have never put on so many splints, plasters, slings and bandages all in one go before or since. Eventually the rest of the patients were sorted out and warded, and I was ready to go into theatre. In the meantime, my husband had wandered across to the hospital to find out why I was being such a long time. I said that I only had this one last task ahead of me and then I would be finished. Rex said he would wait in that case and walk home with me. I went into theatre and began.

Suddenly Mallam Manda, the theatre nurse, said to me, "Your husband is watching you" – and sure enough, Rex was looking through the window in the theatre door – I don't think he had ever seen inside an operating theatre before. I made a mental note to ask him not to watch again, because I felt, and still feel, strongly about patient confidentiality, though I understood why Rex was looking – he was watching me and not the patient. I concentrated again on the job in hand.

A few moments later, Mallam Manda said, "Your husband has gone. I don't think he likes it very much." Indeed he had gone – right home without waiting for me, and indeed he didn't 'like it very much'. "How you can do that," he said when I finally arrived back at the house, "I shall never know." I didn't bother after that to ask him not to stay and watch again. I knew any danger of him doing so was now non-existent!

Chapter 20

Although I was not sent out bush touring when in Katsina, I did have one assignment out of station in February 1959 – and what a strange experience that was.

We had been visited by one of our dispensary attendants who worked in a small bush dispensary very near to the border between Nigeria and French Niger. He complained that many 'French' people came across the border to his dispensary, thereby using a great proportion of his supplies of medicines. He pointed out to us that he could only order supplies at certain times, and that he thought they should be used only for patients in his own country. Clearly he felt that the French should look after their own. Could we do something about it?

There was a hospital and a doctor in Maradi, the nearest town to Katsina over the border. It was a place that our expats would visit from time to time for a bit of time off, so it wasn't exactly at the ends of the earth from us. I was told to go over there to see the medical officer and try to resolve the problem. Accordingly a letter was sent to the French doctor to tell him that I would visit (a date was given so that he could expect me), and the nature of the situation was described.

In due course I set out. Rex took some casual leave, in order to accompany me, as neither of us had seen Maradi before. We decided to take our camp kit just in case the visit took longer than expected, and we also took Ali our cook with us. Although we both spoke some Hausa, it was always a good idea to have somebody with you who was fluent in the language, and who was also African. Ali was a help to us in another way too. We had decided that we ought to take some French money with us in case we needed to spend anything for an overnight stay. We could have gone to the local bank – Barclay's Bank DCO. Another option was that I had been told one could get a better rate of exchange in the Katsina market, but I didn't think I had enough command of Hausa to start on that tack. However, Ali told us that he knew a trader in the town who would do an exchange for us. So he took us to his friend's house – one of the mud houses along a small alleyway.

We were admitted to his house, taken through all sorts of passages and rooms to the inner sanctum, where the trader opened a 'secret' hole in the mud wall and took out bundles of notes with which to make the exchange. I am sure we got it done more cheaply than by going to the bank!

We set off late morning, after I had done my ward rounds, and planned to arrive at the doctor's house round about the end of siesta. The journey itself was quite straightforward except that when we went through the Nigerian border there was a sort of no-man's-land between that and the French border. It was a few miles before we reached the border of Niger, and I wondered which side of the road I should travel on until I reached French territory where I knew I would be driving on the right hand side of the road. African drivers could be rather erratic and I didn't want to find myself arguing with a lorry on the wrong side. The roads were not very wide anyway. In the end I opted for the middle, and tried to judge which side any oncoming driver chose when he saw me, and then I quickly swerved to the other. Luckily the road was straight so that we all saw one another in good time, and the ploy worked.

At one point, as we were going along just before we reached the Nigerian border, we came across a line of men walking towards Katsina, all carrying huge head loads. I said to Ali, "They will all be very tired by the time they get to Katsina with those loads".

"They are not going to Katsina," replied Ali, "They are going to Maradi like we are."

"But they're going the wrong way," I said.

"No, Madam," said Ali "They will turn round soon. If they go on our road, they will soon come to policemen who will look at their loads and make them pay money to take them to Maradi. They are going to a place they know where there are no policemen so that they can go to Maradi without having to pay." Voila! Luckily the Douane didn't seem to be interested in us – the barrier was quickly lifted and we were waved through.

Eventually, after our arrival in Maradi, we managed to find the doctor's house. His steward told us that we were not expected and that the doctor was in siesta and could not be disturbed.

We waited.

Eventually a rather not-best-pleased doctor came through to see us. He spoke neither English nor Hausa. It appeared that the French expected the local people in their colonies to learn to speak French rather than themselves learning how to speak local languages as we did. We spoke some Hausa but only the French that we remembered from our school days. By dint of the doctor speaking (in French) to his steward, who spoke to Ali (in Hausa), who in turn spoke to us (in English), and vice versa, we managed to get the message across about the use of our dispensary over the border. We gathered from all the interpretation which went on that the doctor was in fact shrugging his shoulders and saying, "How can I stop people going to your clinics?" I suppose he couldn't really, but he wasn't being very helpful about it, for he didn't seem inclined to talk it over and see if between us we couldn't come up with some ideas to lighten the situation. They didn't seem to have any system of dispensaries as we did anyway.

In fact, he told us that, in his view, the French colonial government in Niger treated the civilians as second class citizens. Almost all the resources, he said, went to the military, leaving very little for any public services, including hospitals. And no, he had not had any letter from me. It would have gone from Nigeria to the coast and had not yet come up country to him. He softened up a bit as he spoke, and offered to show us round his hospital. It looked a lot cleaner in a way than ours – I think because of the white tiling which went halfway up the walls in the wards, which gave a good impression. I had the feeling that our hospital was rather bigger but that his had nicer buildings.

That all done, we broached the subject of an overnight stay. Was there anywhere that we could get a bed for the night? Clearly he was not at all inclined to offer us hospitality himself – that was never suggested. How different from us all in Nigeria where any expatriate would have been only too keen to have visitors – they provided something new and different, and fresh conversation. If nothing else, one always offered a cool drink. He hummed and ha'd and finally suggested "L'Encampment".

"What is that?" we asked.

He indicated that he would lead us there in his car and that we should follow him. We did – or at least tried to. We were in my car and I was driving, (I always seemed to be the one driving if ever we were in awkward situations!). He drove at about a million miles an hour, or so it seemed, and there was I trying to follow the cloud of dust he stirred up in front of me, while driving on an unaccustomed side of the road hoping to avoid the other cars and drivers who were also going at breakneck speed all over the place. Luckily we arrived without mishap at 'L'Encampment.'

The doctor then spoke rapidly to a large French lady who seemed to be in charge, and then within seconds he had gone and left us to our fate.

And in a way, fate it was. She, although quite friendly, was clearly trying to make me understand that she had no rooms at all.

We were standing on a long verandah with rooms – or at least, doors, off it at frequent intervals, which we imagined led to rooms. I was trying to make out what she was saying when she suddenly grabbed my hand and pulled me towards one of these doors. "Venez!" she exclaimed, and flung open the door, then pulled me back just as I was about to go through it. A good thing she did, because although it did indeed lead into a room, it was a room with no floor but just a hole of uncertain depth. Rapidly she showed me into the others – all the same. Then she indicated that if we wished, we could put up our camp beds (if we had any – she had none!) at the far end

175

of the verandah, and we were welcome to do that for one night. And that is what we did. We were glad at any rate that we had packed our camping kit, including mosquito nets.

Then she said there was no food – sorry.

No, she said, there was nowhere that Ali could go to buy food for us all either. And the latrines were out at the back.

All we had with us was a tiny amount of squash left in our flasks and the remains of our lunchtime sandwiches. So we set up our beds, had a grand supper out of what was left of our lunch (I think it was one sandwich and a hardboiled egg actually), and more or less turned in for the night. Ali meantime had been told that he must join the other 'boys' out back.

We hadn't been asleep for more than a couple of hours before we were woken up by the sounds of a large vehicle driving into the compound. Seconds later we heard Madame greeting the driver loudly and with great pleasure. Later still we heard the unmistakeable sounds of food being served and eaten with relish. Glasses clinked, plates rattled, and it seemed as if almost a party was going on. Finally it all settled down and quietness reigned. We went back to sleep – but only for the same thing to happen again some time later on.

I don't know how many times this happened again during the night, but Madame hardly seemed to sleep, and food and drink were served time and time again. We wondered if L'Encampment was perhaps a pull in café and doss-house for long distance lorry drivers coming in off the Sahara. Ordinary people like us were definitely out of place there. We were very glad when morning came and we could pack up and go. Before setting off we both visited 'out back' for the loo. I never saw such chaos and filth as there was out there. It was the worst and dirtiest place I think I have ever come across. Ali, who had been unceremoniously sent there to find himself somewhere to sleep for the night was disgusted and said he didn't know how the boys who worked there stayed, it was so bad. I don't know to this day why they were not all decimated with dysentery and more.

We were very thankful to get back to Katsina.

Once again we were taken by Ali to the house of his friend the trader who gave us back our English money and took back his French notes, of which we had spent precisely nothing. I think he must have been a very old friend of Ali's, for he didn't want any commission from us at all – we found that most unusual.

I have said that most of the houses in Katsina itself were built of mud and that the walls of the town were also made of mud. Government accommodation, by and large, was built with breezeblocks. However, a few of the Senior

Service houses on the GRA were made of mud and must therefore have been pretty old and built long before the days of breeze blocks. When Rex had been in Katsina some years before we met, he had lived in one of these big mud houses. There is only a tiny snapshot of it in our photograph album but you can see what it was like. He said that it was all right in the hot season, and so long as one was fit and well, but in the rains it could be gloomy and could leak; and if you were ill it was not very nice either. He had suffered from jaundice while he was there and had been in his mud house for some time before being taken to hospital in Kano, so he knew. Also, he said, in the hot season, many people would take their beds out onto the flat roofs of such houses, and sleep outside for coolness. But when he took his bed up onto his roof, he found that a group of vultures also frequented it, which made it not such a good proposition for him, for apart from the noise there was the problem of being dive bombed with their droppings. So he went back inside and suffered the heat.

However, such houses were a bit of colonial history, and very interesting. We stayed in one once on our return from leave, until our own house had been opened up for us again. With huge high rooms and whitewashed walls, and with their roofed verandahs with archways and columns through which one overlooked the compound, and with the verandahs being also whitewashed inside, these houses were fascinating to be in.

Another special occasion that I remember in Katsina was when an afternoon of polo, followed the next morning by a huge durbar, had been arranged by the Emir. All this was in aid of a film company who must have been making a documentary about Nigeria. The polo matches played were as fast as ever. I felt quite sorry for the cameraman because he had to stand by his camera no matter what, while the other chaps with him could dodge out of the way (and did, very smartly) when a bunch of horses came full pelt towards them, often just at a moment when their riders were swinging their polo sticks. However, nobody was knocked over and I suppose it could be said that a good time was had by all, cameraman included.

The next morning was far more un-nerving for the filming team. Not at first, for the first part of the durbar was really quite quiet and dignified. As usual, there was a small dais put up in front of the palace, where various senior service personnel and Native Authority officials were allocated seats. Rex and I, and a friend who was also at the college, were there as official guests, both men dressed in their tropical weight suits as it was a formal event. I probably wore my hat and stockings likewise.

In front of the dais was the local Dandal Way – a huge empty area stretching a long way ahead, bounded eventually by buildings of one sort and another. From the far corner of this area came all the district heads and their retinues, as had been the case in Maiduguri, progressing at first slowly, with jesters preceding them, and with retainers on foot surrounding them. All were dressed in colourful flowing robes and it was a great sight. When all the chiefs had gone past, there was a long line of Native Authority Police, in their blue uniforms and red fezzes, followed in turn by a line of warders from the prison, again all in their matching uniforms and caps.

Once they had gone by, a line of horses, covered in brilliant trappings, and each led by a groom, proceeded along the same route up to the dais, thence being taken through a big archway into the palace compound. These represented the finest horses from the Emir's stables.

After the horses came camels, also caparisoned in bright cloths, ridden by men who beat huge drums – rather like we see the great drum horses at our Trooping the Colour ceremony. They too, entered the palace compound.

Finally, we saw one last horse coming along, decorated with harness even more lavish than the others, and we saw that the rider was shaded by a huge brilliantly coloured parasol, held by a man walking alongside the animal. This rider could only be one person – the Emir himself, robed and turbaned – and veiled as befitted a man who lived near the desert. Trumpeters accompanied him too, sounding fanfares as he rode, and outriders surrounded him – several of them being dogari – the Emir's personal messengers, in robes of dark green and scarlet.

Once arrived at the dais, he dismounted and took his seat.

So far, so good. The cameramen were standing just in front of the dais, and their cameras had been turning all the time. They would have got some good pictures. But, although I am sure they would have been told what to expect, they were completely unprepared for the impact of the next stage – that of the horsemen who, in a long line across the Dandal, came at full gallop, at breakneck speed, waving their spears high above their heads in salutes to the Emir, right up to the film crew, when they suddenly reined in their horses within inches, and stopped, pulling the animals back on their haunches and raising clouds of sand in the process. The cameramen dived for cover when they saw the line of galloping beasts, not caring what became of their cameras!

The riders had therefore to go back and do it all over again. Again the camera crew jumped for their lives. The whole thing had to be repeated four or five times before they were brave enough and confident enough to stay put and film while these lines of men all but enveloped them. I think that in the end they would have got some quite dramatic pictures.

The crowds always get very excited on occasions like these, and near us they were being controlled by Native Authority policemen with whips. The whips didn't really hurt – indeed when I was at one of the Agricultural shows in Maiduguri, and, together with others had got rather near to a bull that was charging up the arena, I received my lash too as the policemen tried to move us away. It just reminded us that we should move, that was all. It wasn't painful.

After it was all over, the Emir once again mounted his horse and rode into his compound, preceded as before by all the procession, horsemen, camels, all the men on foot, and the whole thing finished.

Rex, Bill and I, who had walked from our houses, then walked back home. It was by now almost mid day and very hot indeed. I don't know how the two chaps coped with their suits because I found it overpowering even in a cotton dress. As we walked, the townspeople were also drifting off to their houses – up alleyways, through little entrances in the walls, and along the larger roads, while the sun and heat were reflected off the red-gold mud walls and off the road underfoot. We were in the midst of a crowd of people, children, horses, goats, sheep, occasional donkeys, everyone and everything. And I still have the cine film I took that morning, though after so many years it is getting a bit weary and losing some colour.

The sand was so hot to walk on that it would have been difficult for somebody like me to walk barefoot – I would have burnt my feet in no time. The Africans, most of whom did go barefoot, developed thick hard skin, as hard as leather, on the soles of their feet, and didn't seem to notice the heat. I remember once that a Lebanese man who had been sent to the local prison for some reason, was brought to me by a warder because he had asked for permission to wear sandals. He said, and I could understand it, that his soft-skinned feet were so painful with the hot surfaces over which he had to go that he could hardly bear to walk. The warders were rather contemptuous of this request, saying that as a prisoner he could not have any privileges. It took quite a lot of explaining to make them understand that he was not asking for privileges but that he was really getting his feet badly burnt.

One reason why so many people got hookworm was because of walking barefoot. Few, if any, would be aware of the life cycle of the hookworm among the local populace, and anyway shoes or sandals cost money. People had always walked barefoot and always would do. Although it was a status symbol to own a pair of football boots if you were a student, most would take their boots off for preference when playing simply because they were not accustomed to footwear of any kind.

One nice thing about the Katsina Club (a much smaller club than that in Maiduguri, but then we were a much smaller station) was that somebody had organised a tiny kitchen garden which was supervised by a European.

It meant that two or three times a week, when things were in season, we could buy fresh produce. When we first arrived, all we could get amounted to one tiny lettuce and a handful of runner beans. Later on we were able to have cauliflower and cabbage, a great treat. In Maiduguri, even potatoes were just about unheard of. What we got in Katsina was like having ambrosia. Otherwise, you managed with what scarce supplies might be in the market – tomatoes or peppers, and tinned goods from the canteens. In Katsina there was only one canteen up near the GRA. There was no system there like the present day supermarkets. You had to ask for one item at a time and if it was in stock, the counter hand would get it before you asked for the next thing you wanted. It took a long time to complete your order for the week. I was reminded of going to the shops for my mother when I was a child.

Although our compound in Katsina was large, it was impossible to do anything about growing flowers or vegetables. Despite my best efforts the most I ever managed to grow was a couple of carrots! Why? Well, our compound had fence posts but there was no fence. It had a gateway but no gate. Up on the GRA this would not have mattered, but where we were in the African town, it mattered a lot because as a result the compound was constantly occupied by goats and donkeys. The goats were insatiable, eating anything and everything and even trying to steal food from each other's mouths. Often they succeeded. In the dry season, when nothing really grew, they went to all sorts of lengths to find something green. Some had learnt to walk to a small thin sapling and bend it over by walking along with near and offside legs on either side of it. They simply walked right along it, bending it until they reached the top of it when they would eat the tiny leaves there which other goats had not been tall enough to get to. They loitered especially round our kitchen door, realising that there was food inside. Occasionally Ali would have to chase a goat out of the kitchen where it had started to nose around to see what it could find. Goats were really quite intelligent. Not so the donkeys. I wrote to my parents:

'T.T.C.
Katsina
Northern Nigeria
11.11.58

The goats are a problem, they get in everywhere and are cute enough to do it very quietly... Also the donkeys are a nuisance for getting into the compound, but they are terribly stupid...You can be roaring along the road in your car, and a donkey will stand in the middle of the road and look at you and practically fall asleep... All the other animals, even the sheep, which are also very stupid, will get out of the way eventually, but never the donkeys.'

The only time when I knew donkeys to be frisky was one night (in Katsina) after we had gone to bed. We were suddenly woken up by a great noise of braying, together with much thudding and banging, some of which was against the glass doors opening from our bedroom to the compound.

We discovered that two donkeys were having a fight to the death just outside the bedroom. What if they broke the glass, or worse, the whole doors and fell into the room, we wondered. We lay there holding our breath, and in the end they must have decided that they had settled whatever argument they had, and they departed. Luckily no glass was broken, though it was surprising in view of the tremendous bangs and thuds against the doors!

My work continued as usual – nothing new to report there. When I had arrived in Katsina there had been two medical officers, but one was due to go on leave. So my time was taken up with working just as much as it had been in Maiduguri.

We made friends, both African and European, and were therefore soon in the throes of entertaining and being entertained. It was difficult for us to go out in the evenings actually because very few houses had telephones, and I was always liable to be called to the hospital. The GRA was a mile or two from the town where we lived, so I couldn't leave Ali to answer the phone and come to get me if I was needed as I had sometimes done in Maiduguri. It was therefore better for us to have people in to our house. Both Rex and I were extremely busy in our respective jobs, so much so that there were times when we hardly saw one another, particularly when the College Principal was away and Rex had to act for him in addition to everything else. At such times the few evenings we could spend at home, just the two of us, were very special.

Next door to us, just across the road, was a mud compound where the (African) Native Authority Visiting Teacher and Councillor for Education, Mallam Hassan, lived with his family. He had known Rex previously, and would come across to us sometimes in the evening for a chat and a cool drink. He had welcomed me to Katsina and had invited me to his compound to meet his household. I would often see the wives outside during the day, pounding corn in huge pestles ready for making their meals. I would also see them threshing corn. There would be a great pile of it on the ground outside the compound, and two or three would beat it with flails, after which others would gather handfuls into large round trays, shaking them from side to side. As they shook, the husks would fly off and presumably what was left would be the grain that they would use. Very time consuming and tiring too, I think. But it was a simple way of doing it, which must have gone on from time immemorial.

I was delighted when an invitation came to me one day to go over to attend a party that the wives were holding to celebrate the naming of a new baby in the household. There was no invitation for Rex, as men were not allowed to see this part of the festivities. People had been arriving for the event for several days beforehand. I was told that the Imam would give the child its name in the morning (men were allowed to be present for that part of the ritual), and the festivities would be inside the compound in the afternoon, when all men would be banished until the evening.

When I arrived at the appointed time, I found the compound to be full to capacity with women, young and old, all dressed in their best. Everyone was happy and excited, conversation flew back and forth in a great chatter. The new mother and the baby were seated at one end, the baby lying on a large cushion and fast asleep, remaining asleep the whole time too.

During the afternoon, several of the older women seated themselves in a circle on the ground, with huge upturned calabashes on their knees. These they used as drums, beating all kinds of fascinating rhythms with their hands on the curved surfaces, while two younger women, colourfully dressed, danced in the middle. When the dance ended, the other guests pressed coins onto the foreheads of the dancers in appreciation. This all went on for some time, and seemed to be the main part of the celebrations. I had taken my cine-camera with me and managed to catch just a few seconds of the goings-on. It was all rather dark inside the compound walls, but even so a little of the scene did come through.

A week or so later, Mallam Hassan was over at our house. The developed film had just been returned to me that day, so I put it through the projector for him. He shot out of his chair, dashing right up to the wall against which the film was projected.

"I have never seen this myself!!!" he exclaimed.

He had never had any idea what went on at such times during the women's party, and was tickled to death to see even a few seconds of it. I guess it gave him quite a bit of kudos among his friends.

Christmas 1958 approached, and I resurrected my tiny tree with the equally tiny baubles that I'd used the previous year. After some pressure from my husband, I managed to get hold of some crepe paper and made a few paper chains for the lounge as well. It was seasonably 'cold' too, being Harmattan again. The temperature in the house had dropped to about 60 degrees F in the early mornings, and I would wear a cardigan for work first thing. It still warmed up during the day, but the nights could be very cold. Everyone in station made an effort for Christmas – there was a carol evening at the Residency and there was an extra Open Night at the club, as well as the customary party complete with Santa Claus for the children. For New Year there was to be a fancy dress party at the club as well. Everyone tried to have at least one day off to go to Kano for Christmas shopping. The 200 mile round trip didn't seem to be any big deal – with so little traffic and a not-too-bad tarmac road (except for the potholes) you could get a bit of speed up and do the distance between Katsina and Kano in about two or two and a half hours. It would have been a different story had the road been laterite as at Maiduguri.

Kano was our 'bright lights' city. There were decent canteens – you could even buy furniture and clothes there; and there was the well-run air conditioned Central Hotel for meals and if wanted, an overnight stay, as well as the Airport Hotel and restaurant, which was a popular place to go to for an evening meal. You could sit there and watch the planes come and go, marvelling that in just a few hours (10 hours then) the plane you saw take off would be in London, and the people you saw embarking would be on their way to their families, and living in houses where you could drink water straight from the taps. They could run baths directly – hot ones too, instead of having the water heated up in a zinc bucket on an outside wood fired stove. And for people from outlying bush stations there would also be the luxury of electric light instead of Tilley lamps and candles. How wonderfully such contrasts succeed in making life interesting and full.

We got all our Christmas shopping done, and on return home organised a Christmas dinner party to which we invited as many people as we could think of who would be on their own otherwise – single people, and those whose families were not out with them. We planned to use the remains of the lower tier of our wedding cake as a Christmas cake, setting the top tier aside for our families back home.

This top tier posed a slight problem for us – that of weight, for we would be flying home when we went on leave. Already I was trying to work out what we could safely leave in Nigeria in the way of clothes and incidental belongings, for I knew that we would be buying new things when on leave, to replenish and extend our wardrobes. I also knew that I wanted to carry both my cine-camera and projector back to the UK so that they could be serviced and cleaned. Both seemed to be full of dead insects!

A solution to the problem suddenly presented itself in the shape of one of the VIPs from Kaduna who came to Katsina and who stayed with us for a few days – he was one of the senior medical officers at headquarters and I had met him when I was in Kaduna myself on the Leprosy course there. He was due to go on leave shortly. "We're going by sea this time for a change," he said to me. "Give your cake to me and we'll take it with us. If you give me your parents' address, I'll post it to them after I get home." He and his family lived in Edinburgh.

Our wedding cake would probably originally have been exported from the UK to Lagos by sea. From there it had been carried as air freight north to Maiduguri for our wedding, a distance of about a thousand miles. Following the wedding, we had taken it with us from Maiduguri to Katsina by car. Now the top tier would be driven from Katsina to Kaduna and thence either by car or by air to Lagos. From Lagos it would be transported by sea to a south coast UK port – a fortnight's voyage. Then it would be carried on the long train trip to Edinburgh, from where, finally, it would be posted to Hull – journeying no doubt on a mail train. I often think it must have been the most travelled wedding cake in the world!

Eventually, in early 1959, the time came for our own leave. I had arranged to stop working about ten days before we left in order to pack up the household. Every time one went on leave, one's own possessions had to be packed up and put into store with the Public Works Department. This was because there was never any guarantee that you would be posted back into your previous station – you could well be posted elsewhere, so that your loads would have to be sent off to your new base. And anyway, somebody would be sent to replace you while you were out of the country, and whoever it was would be living in your house, and would have all their own things with them. Because I was now a married woman, I had to resign each time my husband went on leave. On return I had to apply for a work permit again before I could be re-employed as a temporary officer.

This time, Rex had five months' leave owing, so that we had a very long spell in the UK. After that, and so long as he was posted to an educational institution, he would have to take an annual leave to fit in with the academic year. That meant that we would get three months away from Nigeria. You had one week of leave for every month worked, plus an extra two weeks if you travelled each way by air, to make up for the time people had extra if they sailed home. For all other jobs in education, and for other professions, leave entitlements were calculated on the basis of your age. Up to a certain age, your tour of duty was 18 months, as mine would have been had I not married. After a certain age (about 40, I think, though I stand to be corrected on that), your tour would be 15 months, and after another age milestone, you only worked for a year before going on leave.

We were posted back to Katsina in September 1959 on return from our long break, but I did not resume work at first, as I was by then pregnant, and felt that it might be wise to take life easily until the baby had arrived. I

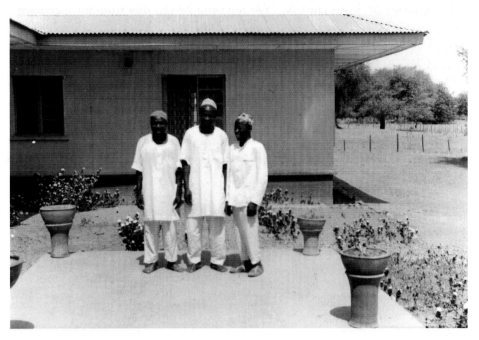

Our houseboys outside our Katsina house.
Left to right: Audu (steward), Ali (headboy and cook), Momso (small boy).

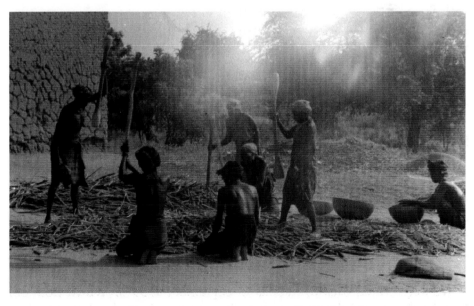

Our next door neighbours winnowing corn outside their house, Katsina.

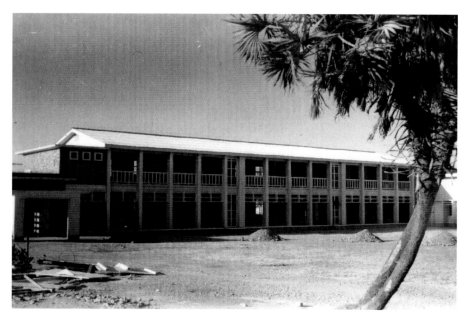

One of the new buildings at Katsina Teacher Training College, Katsina, 1958.

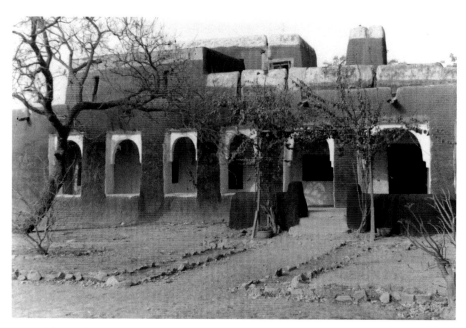

An old mud built Senior Service house, Katsina.

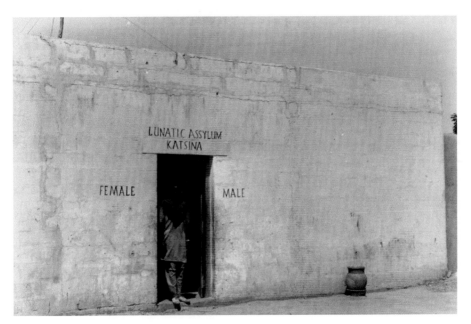

Entrance to the Lunatic Asylum, Katsina.

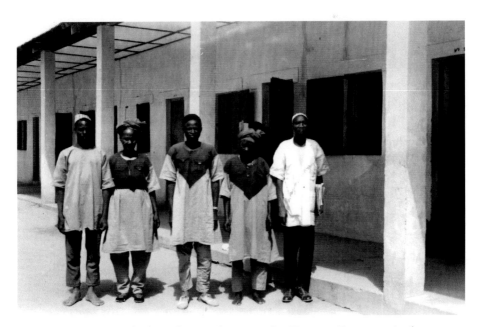

Nurse (in white jacket) and attendants at the Katsina Lunatic Asylum.

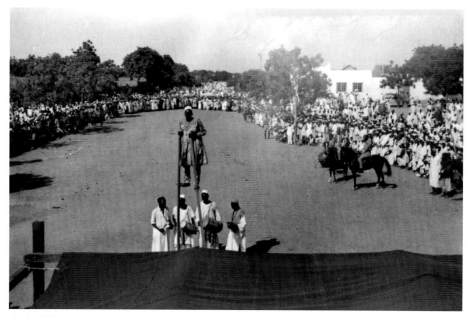

Stilt walker entertaining the Emir of Daura and the crowd at a durbar in Daura, 1958.

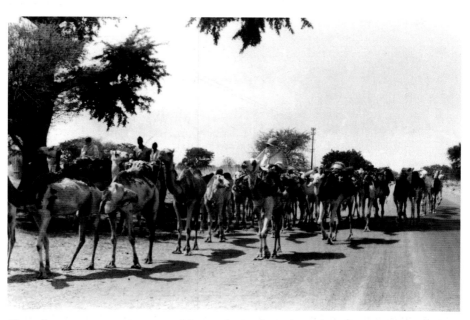

Camel caravan coming into Kano along the Kano-Katsina Road.

was soon very bored with nothing to do though, and was therefore delighted when the medical officer in charge at the hospital asked me if I would do a sort of locum there for a few weeks as he was short of a doctor. Would I indeed! Most certainly I would, and wrote to my parents that I felt as if I had come alive once more. It was great to be working again if only for a limited time. In addition to that I was on tap for other things. The Katsina Training College and the Government Girls' School Principals asked me if I would give a course of First Aid Classes at both places, as they felt this would be useful to the students in their future careers. I sorted out a series of talks and practical sessions, and attended each place weekly. Everyone applied themselves well and I was pleased with the way things went, until one day I saw that the girls were quite deliberately taking no notice of anything I said. Some sat and looked out of the window. Others fidgeted and talked to each other. Not one volunteered, as they usually did eagerly, to demonstrate particular practical tasks. This was totally out of character and I couldn't understand it at all. They had all been so keen and deft until then. Anyway, I persevered until the end of the session. Afterwards I told the Principal how odd their behaviour had been and how I was at a loss to make anything of it.

A few days later she had found out what it was all about. It seemed that during the lecture previous to the one where nobody had worked, I had congratulated the girls on their excellence at the practical items such as bandaging, putting on slings and so on. I had added jokingly, "You'd all make wonderful nurses."

The girls had decided, because of that last remark, that there was an ulterior motive in the First Aid course, which was that secretly there were plans to train them all as nurses. Since they all wanted to be married when they left school, as tradition demanded, they determined that the only way not to finish up being nurses would be to do so badly in the assessment at the end of the course that we would think they were hopeless and would give up on them. None of them put any effort into their First Aid from that moment onwards in spite of everything that we said.

Tradition was very strong, as indeed it should be – nobody wants to lose their own culture. However I feel that people should be willing to add new and useful knowledge to what they already have and this can be done without destroying cultural traditions, surely. And what about their households when they did marry? None of them had thought how useful their teaching could have been in that context. A pity.

Anyhow, what with my short locum, and my teaching duties, together with my willingness to be escort for any patient who needed to be taken to hospital in Kano (something that I did on occasion), I managed to pass the months before the birth of our baby quite pleasantly after all.

185

It may be of interest to know how my pregnancy and delivery were managed and monitored in Nigeria. Many expatriate wives, if they became pregnant, were sent back to their own country for the last few months and for the delivery, while others might be sent to big centres where there were more facilities, at least a month in advance of the expected date of delivery – Kano, Lagos and so on. I was lucky in that I was pretty fit, and because our station was so near to Kano where there was actually a specialist obstetrician, Kay Drury, I was, therefore, allowed to stay in Nigeria for the delivery, and what is more, Kay told me that because I was so well, and because she knew that my husband could down tools if necessary and drive me to Kano in a matter of not much longer than a couple of hours, she would let me stay in Katsina until only two weeks before the babe was due. She asked me to go to Kano to see her every month, while getting the Katsina MO to have a look at me halfway between my Kano visits. In this way somebody would monitor me every two weeks, so that any problem could be quickly picked up and I could if need be, get to Kano quickly and early.

How well I remember those trips to Kano. We would get up at about half past four in the morning, when, during Harmattan, it was very cold. We would be wrapped up in sweaters and cardigans as we set off, over the bumpy road – perhaps it seemed bumpier to me than it was, but I didn't enjoy those journeys much. As daylight gradually came, we would see the occasional person on the side of the road in villages that we passed through. Everyone would be huddled up somehow – caftans or other garments wrapped round them tightly as they tried to keep warm.

And how good it was when we arrived at the Central Hotel where we would make our base for the day, starting with breakfast before going to the hospital to see Kay. She was a lovely person and worked extremely hard. Often she looked very tired, and we were pleased when we managed to persuade her to come and stay with us for a weekend, when we set out to look after her and make sure she was idle while she was with us.

I found that one of the nursing sisters who had been in Maiduguri with me (she of the special wedding cake knife) – was now in charge at the Nassarawa Hospital in Kano. She very kindly offered to put me up for the last fortnight of pregnancy when I had to be in Kano. Kate Griffin was kindness itself and did her best to help the time to pass pleasantly for me.

Our baby was actually due on Christmas Day. Rex was both looking forward to its arrival, and dreading it too, for in Katsina, the person who had to take the part of Santa Claus for the Club children's party was always the newest father on the station. Every year, Santa had to use a different form of transport, and this time he was to ride in on a camel. As I have said somewhere earlier in this account, the last and only four-legged creature

Rex had ever bestridden was a seaside donkey when he was a child. He was horrified at the idea of a camel – they really did seem to be so far from the ground!

He was lucky, because our daughter came into the world on Christmas Eve, and by the time the news spread, he was safely back in Kano. The next newest father had to take on the role of Santa at short notice (I wonder what he thought to that) – and we were told later that as luck had it, the saddle slipped and he fell off his mount. So far as I know he was not hurt, but I can record that my husband was mightily relieved to have been a hundred miles away!

Santa Claus had some odd adventures in regard to his transport in Northern Nigeria, and I imagine many people could produce amusing tales in that respect. When it was my first Christmas in Nigeria, Santa in Maiduguri was to arrive on an ox-cart. They didn't seem to know about snow and sleighs and reindeer in the tropics. All the children were waiting at the club – and waiting – and waiting. No Santa Claus arrived at the appointed time, and I'm sure several children must have thought he had forgotten them so far from their own countries. Then at last, a very weary Santa turned up, hot in his robes and extremely tired. It seemed that en route he was stopped by a keen Native Authority policeman – somebody who had no idea what the red robes and white beard meant, much less the sacks of parcels. All the policeman was concerned about was the fact that a local bye-law stated that nobody was to ride in an oxcart – any person with the cart should walk and only goods could be in it. Santa, therefore, was required to accompany the policeman to the police station to explain himself before being allowed (presumably with a caution) to walk all the way from there to the GRA and the Senior Service Club, leading the ox which pulled the cart and the sacks of presents. Santa didn't dare to remove his costume in case any of the children saw that he was only somebody's Dad! However, he performed his duty satisfactorily, but not until he had downed about a gallon of fluid and rehydrated himself!

I had a lot of visitors before I was allowed to leave Nassarawa Hospital and go home, among them the Senior Medical Officer (Kano). He and his wife came to see me, bringing with them an enormous bunch of roses from their compound, a rare gift out there, and they were lovely. While we were chatting, he suddenly said to me, "The Emir of Katsina has put in a special request that you should remain in Katsina. He has appreciated the fact that at last there is a lady doctor and therefore somebody who can see his wives. The wives like it too. Because of his request, and if you agree to stay, we would approach Education Ministry to ask if they would agree to keep your husband in Katsina at the college so that you would not be separated."

I was very much touched to think that the little I had done in the wives' compound had been well thought of. However, I knew that I was not prepared to do anything which might affect Rex's career in any way. I didn't want to be the means of his having to stay in Katsina and perhaps miss out on some other posting, and said so. So, no, I finished up, I couldn't agree to the offer, though I appreciated it. "I told you that's what she'd say," put in his wife with a smile, "and it's what I would have said too." And that was that.

The time came for me to return to Katsina with our daughter. The boys were waiting outside the door as we drove into the compound. They all shook hands with us both (a handshake was an important gesture), and Ali looked at me and said "Madam go young again". They admired the baby (even though she was a girl and not a son), and our family life began.

One last thing to record about the birth was that the Emir's number two polo team mate, whom I have mentioned before, came to our house a day or so after my return, asking to see me and to admire the child. This again was quite something because several Africans we knew had, Rex said, been a bit exercised as to whether to congratulate him or commiserate with him because our daughter was not a boy.

Having paid his compliments to us both, our visitor then said that he had brought a gift for the baby, and to our amazement produced his own personal replica of the Nigeria Polo Association Georgian Cup that the Katsina team had won in 1958. We couldn't believe that he had wanted to part with so important an object, but he was adamant – it was for this new baby. We thought that was a lovely gesture.

Chapter 21

Towards the end of May 1960 the time for our next leave arrived. As we packed up our personal chattels for storage we wondered if, at the end of our leave, we would be unpacking them in the same house, or if Rex would be posted elsewhere. Several possibilities of alternative placements had already been suggested to him but no decision had been made. Now, shortly before our return to Nigeria in September 1960 we were surprised and delighted to learn that we were to return to Maiduguri.

A new teacher training college was being started up, this time for men, and Rex was to take charge of it. The first class had just been got together, and a temporary schedule organised, but that was all. The college as yet had no accommodation of its own and that first class of thirty students was housed in a disused building which had once been a Junior Primary School, the Lamisula Junior Primary School. It was a mile or so outside Maiduguri town, along a tree bordered sandy road then called The Avenue of the Sudan. Eventually, we were told, new college buildings would be erected along the airport road, next door to the equally new Provincial Boys' Secondary School, which was being built first. On the other side of the college site was the newly built Government Craft School, so that when everything was done, the airport road would have three education campuses on it.

To our surprise we were put into my old house in Hewby Avenue on the GRA. It was rather nice to be in such familiar surroundings again, and also it was good still to have the privilege of a telephone. We had had one in Katsina which had been essential for both of us because of the nature of our work.

As I have said before, few people then had phones in their houses. For the time being, however, we didn't actually need one – I was not yet working again, and the 'college' in its decrepit school buildings didn't have anything like a telephone. Although people who lived in 'big' places like Jos or Kano could make international calls by that time, we still couldn't do anything like that in Maiduguri. No question of being able to 'phone home', like ET.

For the moment I had not applied for a work permit, feeling that I should concentrate on our infant, though I hoped that before too long I might manage something. Expatriate wives who wanted to work for the Education Department and who had children, had to show to the satisfaction of the authorities in Kaduna that adequate arrangements were made for the care of their children before they were employed. No such condition was ever indicated by the Medical Department, but I imposed my own conditions and would not yet think of taking anything on officially.

However, my husband, being as yet the only member of teaching staff, combined with having to do all the administration of a new college which had to grow and be equipped, found that he was working all hours God sent and still barely had time to deal with the paperwork as he was having to teach every period in the week before even thinking of the desk work. He had to organise, apart from anything else, a recruiting drive leading to interviews of would-be students; and he had to work out how to get food supplies, cooks, labourers, uniforms, teaching materials, innumerable things, so that when he did eventually have proper accommodation, everything could slot in quickly and the place could get going.

We wondered how he could get some quiet time in which to deal with all this kind of thing. The solution we came up with was that I would go, as I had done in Katsina, to the 'college' once or twice a week for a couple of hours and give lectures in First Aid, Health and Hygiene, while he brought his 'desk' home and worked at it undisturbed, keeping an eye on our daughter at the same time. We had been given a big playpen for her, and as she was not doing anything more than crawl as yet, it was easy to watch her and work at the same time. I enjoyed my task and my husband appreciated the few hours of peace and quiet, which enabled him to get through a great deal of paper work, much more than he would have done at the 'college'.

The small school building comprised two classrooms, which were separated by a tiny area that had to act as the office. It housed Rex and his clerk, and behind it was a store cupboard where the storekeeper sat, looking after what bit of equipment there was. Outside the office, on the verandah, sat the college messenger, an old soldier, Dungus Banana, who did all sorts of odd jobs. Chiefly he sat and idly pulled the punkah rope that went through a hole in the wall and wafted a huge punkah over Rex and his clerk. How much good it actually did I'm not sure, but hopefully it stirred the air at least.

One of the classrooms was indeed used as a classroom, while the other, supplied with iron bedsteads, was the room where the thirty students lived, ate and slept. Each had a small locker for his possessions. There was an outside kitchen, and the students, who were given a food allowance of money then, bought their own supplies and cooked their own meals. They also kept the small compound well swept and tidy, as well as the inside of the building. There was no electricity or running water, and they used candles or Tilley lamps, and drew water from a local standpipe. At that time they had no college uniform either but wore their own clothes.

As they were a mile or two out of town, we were a bit anxious in case any of them should be unwell between the time when Rex left college for the day and the next morning, so I formed the routine of going along there in the evenings to make sure that everyone was all right. The head student, Ilyasu Potiskum, was a steady sort of lad, and I took the chance of leaving a small supply of aspirin, Nivaquin (for malaria) and bandages with him, all to be kept in a locked box of which only he held a key, and I told him how and when these should be used in case of any emergency. We couldn't do more than that, but at least it was something. We hoped it would prevent students from possibly wandering off to the hospital if they were not well at night, as we felt responsible for their welfare and they had no means of contacting us for any emergency. When I visited in the evenings, I held in effect a small clinic for any who were under the weather.

I said before that one never knew what one might see on roads, and in Maiduguri there was an ostrich which seemed to wander about all over the place. I would wonder if it had a family anywhere near or if it was a solitary bird. It even appeared on the new college campus once. However, I saw it a few times trailing about the Avenue of the Sudan, and on one memorable occasion it walked in the middle of the road, just as I was driving back home from my teaching session. The ostrich didn't think about dodging onto the side of the road and letting me pass, but instead began to run in front of me. The Avenue of the Sudan was a long road, and the bird ran faster and faster, and I saw from my speedometer that it eventually hit what seemed like an impossible mph before it nipped off the road and into the trees.

The little school had not been used for some time before our students were put into it, and was not in a state of very good maintenance. One day when I was teaching there, I kept thinking to myself, 'The ceiling looks very low – why haven't I noticed this before?' However I finished my session and went back home. Some time later a message came to us to say that the ceiling in that classroom had collapsed and had fallen all over the desks. Luckily no student was in the room and therefore nobody had been hurt.

Despite the difficulties the students worked quite hard, and for my part I was particularly pleased when they put on a display of First Aid skills for one of the senior Inspectors of Education who came from Kaduna to see how things were going on.

I have said that there were three Government education establishments along the airport road, all in a line and all having separate campuses. The Craft School, as I understood it, had to be designed and the building of it to some extent supervised by the Education Officer in charge of it. It must have been a big job, and I remember that the officer in question had first built himself a *rumfa* – a grass hut, made of woven grass matting hung onto poles

– so that he could actually live on the site as everything was being erected. The building work included not only all the school buildings dormitories, workshops, kitchens and so on, but also staff houses for senior and junior service personnel. How many education officers have to do that here in the UK?

The Provincial Boys' Secondary School was originally the Yerwa Middle School which was in Maiduguri itself, round the corner from the hospital. As soon as their new buildings were ready, the boys moved into them, leaving the old Middle School buildings empty. These were much better than the Lamisula Junior Primary Scool, and we were delighted, as were our students, when the college was told to move in there. Now the lads had decent classrooms, spacious accommodation, their food provided and cooked for them and, best of all, they had a proper football field. This was a delight needless to say.

They also had electric light and running water. And Rex had a new member of staff posted to him – a young man, Laurie Parker, who was a wonderful standby. He took games and PE as well as teaching academic subjects, and so gave my husband some precious administration time at long last. Moreover, there was now somebody else to discuss things with, bounce ideas off and share extra curricular activities like games. What a difference it made. And what a boon the football field was – admittedly it was all sand and no grass, and the boys preferred to play barefoot, but did that matter? Other games could also be tried out such as volleyball (provided that a net could be got hold of from somewhere).

The college clerk was also replaced at that time. Between the departure of the original clerk and the arrival of the new one, there had been a gap of several weeks during which Rex had tried to cope with all the files himself, not easy as there were no proper places to keep them yet. It just happened that we were down at the new premises one Saturday afternoon when a lorry drew up outside the entrance. In the back of it was a pile of boxes and bundles, together with a man and wife and their family. It was the new clerk, just arriving after a long, tiring and dusty journey from his previous posting. He introduced himself, and Rex welcomed him, saying how glad he (Rex) would be of help because he was having such problems finding his way around the files. He spoke half in fun, hoping to put his new member of staff at ease. But Mr Ita Andem Ewa was never a person to hesitate. He was also extremely conscientious. Quickly and firmly he said, "Leave it to me sir." And he went to one of his bundles from which he pulled out a pack of stickers and page markers, and prepared forthwith to sort out the files. He was to prove to be a wonderful person to have in the office. A serious man, but very kindly, totally efficient, trustworthy and conscientious, Mr Ita would describe anyone of whom he approved as 'a very decent somebody'. We thought Mr Ita was one of the best of all the 'decent somebodies' we had known. He stayed at the college as long as we did, being posted elsewhere not very long after our retirement.

While the college was moving into the old Middle School, work was beginning on the definitive campus up the airport road. Taylor Woodrow was the contractor, and the work went ahead really very quickly. Rex and I would go up there most evenings to see what progress there had been during the day. We were told that the 'Arcon process' was being used – that meant that a huge frame was put up first, on which the roof was laid, and the walls were erected after that. Because of the climate, we were told that the buildings would be 'Mediterranean style' – in other words, a large gap would be left between the top of the walls and the roof, so that air could circulate. It sounded a good idea but proved to be a bad one in fact because when the rains broke, the wind blew water right in through these gaps, so that everything inside got soaked – papers would be ruined and blown about the rooms below, other equipment would be spoilt and so on. All the gaps therefore, including those in the staff houses, which had all been built in the same way, had to be filled up. Our cat, as cats, being curious will do, had, unknown to any of us, got itself into our own roof space when the men were working to close the gaps. It was only later on after they had gone home, that we heard the mewing and realised what had happened. When one remembers that the roofs were all of corrugated metal and that water from the tank in the roof space invariably came out of the taps warm, sometimes even hot, it gives an indication of how unbearable the poor animal would find it when trapped there. We managed in the end to get somebody to release it, but what a carry on that was.

When the houses were pegged out in the sand before building started, we feared that they would all be very small, but appearances were deceptive and they were all really quite spacious. Ours, the Principal's house, was really very big. We had two good-sized bedrooms at one end, where we all slept. There was a roomy separate bedroom with an en suite bathroom and separate shower at the other end of the house. This was really the master's room, it being a house built with Moslem families in mind, but we used it as a guest room. It had its own door to the outside so that any guest we had could be totally independent and come and go as he or she pleased if they had things to do which did not include us. Between the two bedroom ends was a huge lounge/dining room. On one of the long sides were several tall windows and the other long side was taken up with sliding patio doors so that the room could be virtually opened up early in the morning and again at the end of the day when it began to get cooler. At 'our' end of the lounge (that is the end farthest from the guest room) a wing was built at right angles to the general line. This had the bathroom in it and continued with the kitchen, though you could only get into the kitchen by going outside first. Outside the lounge and guest room there was a walled compound, nothing like as large as the compound at our other houses, but it was one that could be made into a nice garden. The wall meant that it would be safe from marauding goats too – a bonus! At the other side of the bathroom/kitchen wing there was another smaller compound where our small boy would hang out the washing, and where the gate to the boys' quarters was. Their quarters were outside the compound itself, but adjoining it. It was into that back compound that we would put our beds in the hot season when we slept outside.

I had taken cuttings from various shrubs and trees from our compound in Hewby Avenue, hoping that something would take and grow at the new house. I was not a gardener but thought I should have a go, and to my surprise they all flourished and we had quite a pretty outlook. We had the smaller plants like coleus and canna lilies and morning glory. What I was particularly delighted about was the fact that I managed to get cuttings of the ornamental trees to take as well – bauhinia, which had a pretty yellow flower; gamboges, with brighter yellow blossoms, several oleanders, and best of all – my favourite because of its lovely scent – frangipani. I also got a Flame of the Forest sapling from the Forestry Department, and that grew well. When we left on retirement, it was getting really quite a good size and was very lovely to look at. A year or two later I tried to grow a paw-paw tree in the back compound. It did produce fruit, but small ones, nothing like those which came from the Southern region. My last attempt was to get (also from our Forestry Department) a small jacaranda sapling, but I had been told that they didn't do well in our dry climate, and that proved to be the case. The poor little jacaranda struggled bravely but never really made any progress. Our garden boy decided that a nice edging to the main part of the garden would be a desirable addition. This he provided by salvaging all the empty lager cans that he could lay hands on, and planting then obliquely along the garden margins. We hadn't the heart to take them up, for to do so would have been a real slap in the face for him, so there they stayed. A talking point, if nothing else.

We didn't have any grass lawn, but instead did what many people did, which was to plant portulaca. This eventually spread all over the spaces not occupied by our shrubs. It had flowers, pinkish-red ones, which opened in the early morning and looked very pretty. They shut down again when the sun got high. portulaca had the nickname of 'Administration Rose' because it was said that it opened early but always closed promptly at noon! All other departments went on working until 2 p.m. I am sure the Admin stayed on duty until then, like the rest of us really, but it was a traditional tease to suggest that they didn't.

We had returned from our leave in September 1960. In October, just a month later, Nigeria became fully independent, and there were great celebrations and festivities all over the country to mark this big event.

Princess Alexandra came to Nigeria to represent the Queen, and after attending the formal ceremony of Independence (in Lagos), she travelled around and attended all sorts of events in many different places. Maiduguri was to be one of the places she visited, and so there was a lot of trouble taken to make her stay memorable, hopefully for her and certainly for everyone else. A huge durbar was arranged as might be imagined – the biggest many of us would have seen. Six thousand horsemen, we were told, were coming in for this from all the outlying districts in Bornu. This was a massive influx of people, for wives and families came in with them. A vast area of bush just outside the town was taken over and made into a large camp where they all stayed. People from the town went out there at the end of each day to see what was going on, for all sorts of entertainments would be in progress then. It was understood that expatriate visitors would also be welcomed, and several of us went along. The organisation had been most efficient. First of all one passed the horse lines, with animals tethered in good army fashion, each with its pile of fodder, all munching away and looking remarkably companiable and docile.

There were *rumfas* and other temporary shelters and kitchens set up as well – these would be very simple, just wood fires and perhaps cut-down kerosene cans to be used as ovens for some forms of cooking. Women were constantly preparing meals, pounding corn, cooking, chattering and some just watching, and their children were running about there too, adding to the noise and excitement. Robed men were walking around, meeting and greeting each other, discussing this and that with many repetitions of '*Ina kwana*', '*Ina gajiya*', with the responses '*Lafiya lau, ba gajiya*' which all meant in effect, 'Hi! How are you?' and, 'I'm fine, thanks, all is well.'

In front of me was a large circle of women dancing hand in hand to keep the circle closed, all colourfully dressed. They were Kanuri women – perhaps from the town, I never discovered. Somebody was playing a little tune, maybe on their kind of flutes or pipes, and it was all very jolly.

As I watched, a couple of the women broke the circle and came to take my hands and draw me in. I thought that was a very warm gesture, and for a few moments I too took part in the dance. I have to say that the dancing was not very awe-inspiring – it mostly seemed to be a way of shuffling round, hand in hand. Perhaps there was a pattern of footwork that I missed, but it didn't seem to matter. We were all laughing and enjoying ourselves. Somebody told me afterwards that only the ladies of the night danced for everyone else – but who cared? It was a happy occasion and good to be asked to join in. I had probably had several of them as patients in my clinics and they would know who I was.

The Princess was to stay in the British Residency. Nicky McClintock was the Resident then, and he and his wife Pam worked very hard indeed during the weeks beforehand to make the Residency as welcoming as possible. I remember that Pam spent hours making new cushion covers for the furniture in the sitting room, and new curtains too, for she said the existing ones were getting rather shabby. She was not herself able to be there in the end, when everything started to happen, and I thought it such a pity that she missed it all.

One or two members of the royal party had to be accommodated elsewhere, but not in the Rest House. They had to be where there were telephones so that they could be called at a moment's notice if necessary. We were asked to host the Nigerian equerry. He was a very pleasant young army officer and fitted in well to our household for the brief time he was with us. He was very anxious all the time in case he might disrupt our normal routine, but of course he didn't. In a country where you never knew who would turn up on your doorstep needing hospitality, and we had several unexpected guests that way, one person who you knew would be coming was an easy visitor to arrange for.

The day of the Princess's arrival was quite exciting, for all the district heads and their retinues turned out in their ceremonial robes and trappings and lined the road from the airport (where she would arrive) right up to the gates of the Residency, a distance of three or four miles. That's a lot of men and animals. Hewby Avenue, where we lived, ran only a few yards before it joined the main road along which the royal procession would come, so just at the end of our road there were horsemen and men and women on foot, all in colourful dress, all twirling fans, fly whisks, whatever, while trumpeters sounded fanfares or anything else they could think of. All these people had been in position since 6 o'clock in the morning, as the Princess was expected to touch down at 10 o'clock. In the event, she didn't arrive until noon because, her equerry told us later, she had asked the pilot to make a detour and fly her over Lake Chad before coming in to Maiduguri. How those men and women managed to stay in the burning sun for so long I can't imagine – they must have been broiled in their voluminous robes with no chance of anything to drink. And the horses too – for most of them were caparisoned like those in medieval times, with brilliantly coloured cloths all over them, some quilted, and many of them with elaborate metal harness. I saw broad collars of silver metal (some said to be made of real silver at that), and lots of leather tassels and hangings. Yet men, women and animals remained in place quietly and steadily with no sign of discomfort for six hours. I hoped that Princess Alexandra was properly impressed by what she saw that day because a lot of endurance had gone into the display that she drove past. Nobody had more than a second's glimpse of her as her car flashed by – me included, as I stood next to some of the horsemen, holding six-months old Rosemary in my arms.

The next morning we were all up bright and early for the great durbar. It was a wonderful show – the best, it was said, ever seen in Bornu. Maiduguri did the Princess proud that day.

A reception was also held for her by the Native Authority in their official 'Reading Room' gardens, to which we were both invited. This was a pleasant occasion but very formal. Drinks and 'small chop' (that is canapés and so on) were taken round by stewards. I was talking to a group of Native Authority councillors when a tray of eats was offered to us. We all politely took something. Two of the men I was with bit into what they had taken, decided that they didn't like it and promptly put it back on the tray again before the steward had moved away! I have to admit that I was rather put off accepting any more 'small chop' there.

The order of the day for that party was suits and ties for the men, hats, gloves and stockings for the ladies (expatriates, that is). I had long since given up trying to wear anything with more than a fairly low 'high heel' in Maiduguri because of the sand. However, the Princess had probably not thought or been warned about that. She was brought by car to the venue, and then had to walk through an archway to make her arrival. We were all waiting, and looking towards the archway. She appeared and stood for a moment before starting to walk forwards. As she took the first step, I saw her heels sink right down into the soft sand. She must have dropped about an inch before she recovered herself. I also saw her face just begin to look surprised before she smiled again, and adjusted her pace so that she was almost walking on tip toe to prevent any more sand-sinking. Good for her.

That night, our guest was very late indeed in getting back to our house. When he finally turned up, he sank gratefully into a chair, putting out his hand for the drink that Rex had poured out for him, and said, "I am glad to be here, but forgive me if I don't talk for very long as I want to turn in quickly. We are all so tired, and the Princess wouldn't go to bed! She is enjoying herself too much." 'Too much' in local idiom meant 'very much indeed'.

Chapter 22

During the first few weeks after our return from leave in September 1960, I had been approached by the heads of the Government schools and the Government Women's Training College to ask if I would consider setting up some sort of school medical service. They were all finding that students and pupils lost a lot of lesson time by reporting sick and being sent to the hospital outpatient clinics. This would mean a long walk to the hospital, followed by a long wait to be seen (and adults would push forward in front of youngsters anyway), followed by yet more waiting for lab tests and pharmacy if investigation was needed or medication had to be collected. In addition, girls had to be accompanied by a chaperone, which was not always convenient. Although there was a designated member of staff to whom illness was reported, tutors felt they were not properly competent to diagnose from the often rather odd complaints that were made to them. How was a teacher newly arrived from England, for instance, to know that when a girl told her, "I have a crocodile in my hair" she meant she had nits? If I thought I could do something about this, they said, they would make representation to the Ministry of Education in Kaduna, asking if such an arrangement could be set up with the help of the Ministry of Health.

This whole idea came as a surprise to me. I had not thought of returning to work while our daughter was still in her infancy although I didn't like not working. I gave considerable thought to how such a service might be organised and managed. I had only ever had six months' experience of school medical work, and only at a superficial level really, doing a locum while I waited for my sailing date and my initial departure for Nigeria. How would I set anything up – what background support might I need – all sorts of questions began to come into my mind. And what would I do about my daughter? Rex and I talked the whole thing over very carefully, and I went round the Government educational establishments (all of which were boarding) to discuss things with the Heads there.

Finally I decided that I could organise something on very simple lines, and felt that it was worth a try. If it didn't work out, then I would say so.

Word was sent off to Kaduna, and after a little time I had a letter from the Ministry of Health, in which I was told that I could certainly be employed again, but what I did would depend upon the agreement of the Medical Officer in charge at Maiduguri, who might prefer that I worked as before in the capacity of General Duties MO. I spoke to our MO and explained what

198

had happened, and told him that I was not prepared at that time to go back into the general work that I had done before. I told him how I proposed to arrange a service for the boarding schools, pointing out that it would, in fact, help him anyway because hopefully there would not be the steady flow of students and pupils going to the hospital as hitherto. He would, I argued, benefit from my work even if it was not within the hospital. It was agreed that I should try out the arrangements I had thought of and see how things went.

There was then the question of what facilities and accommodation I could be given at the schools. I visited the lab technician and the pharmacist at the hospital, and explained what I was going to try to do. The lab technician suggested that he would set aside one whole morning each week for the schools work if that would help. It certainly would, and except for anything really urgent, I arranged that any children or students who needed lab investigation should go down first thing in the morning of the appointed day, taking the request slips that I had written. This meant that he could take blood or any other specimens early so that the children could return to school immediately, thus missing as little time as possible from their lessons. I would go down myself at an appropriate time to collect the results of the tests.

The pharmacist likewise agreed to accept prescriptions in my handwriting and to dispense them all at the same time. On my part, I would see that all prescriptions written on any one day were brought to him at one time by some responsible person – a house mother, a teacher perhaps, a school or college messenger maybe, who could wait to collect all the medicines. This meant that no child or student need go to the hospital at all for medicines, again saving lesson time. And I got agreement from the MO in charge that if I deemed somebody to be ill enough for hospital admission I could go ahead with this and start treatment myself without checking with him first.

Next, I had to arrange for suitable accommodation in which to hold my clinics. This school medical service was, as will be realised, going to be very different from that which we know here in Britain. I was going to hold treatment clinics in addition to trying to fit in routine medical examinations. The Provincial Girls' School was able to let me have an empty room in which there would be a table and chairs. This was quite satisfactory, the more so because the room was big enough for me to put up the playpen and put my daughter into it so that she was under my eye all the time. She loved the attention she got from the girls and the housemother who supervised them all, and was as good as gold. My only anxiety had been that she might be exposed to infection, but it seemed that if anyone was really poorly they were kept in bed and I went to the dormitory anyway. The others on the whole seemed to have only minor problems, which were of no risk to her. The

Women's Training College also had a spare room available so we did the same thing there. That too worked out well.

I was already doing an evening 'surgery' at the Men's Training College, so that was not a problem. Later on, when the students moved onto the new campus, I managed to slot them in to my daily schedule without difficulty. At the Provincial Boys' Secondary School, next door to the new Men's college campus, the Principal's wife took my daughter and looked after her together with her own children while I did my clinic there, so that was a happy arrangement for me. Here I was given the use of a classroom store cupboard for my clinics – a big lockable walk-in cupboard/small room, with shelves on which to keep a few basic medicines. We managed to fit into it a small single bedstead at one end so that I could examine the children, and at the other end I had a tiny table and a chair. It was enough.

And finally, one of the staff wives at the Government Craft School, who lived on campus, offered to take my daughter for the time needed, while I conducted my clinic in a small room which served as a dispensary and which was staffed by a real (trained) dispensary attendant. The Craft School only had such a member of staff because he was down on the staff list as a labourer (and probably paid as such) while the Principal of the school managed with one labourer less than his establishment warranted. He had felt, probably rightly so, that the well-being of the schoolboys was more important than a bit of extra labouring help. The appointment was of great help to me too because this man also had an injection licence and could get on with treatment that I prescribed, thus saving me precious time.

As I became more busy with the school work and added duties at the nursing home, I managed to arrange for the Craft School and the Bornu Men's Training College to join up for clinic attendance. Here the services of the Craft School Dispensary Attendant were of great help because he would now give treatments for me in two educational institutions, and he also took prescriptions for both places down to the hospital. Similarly I also arranged for the Provincial Girls' School and the Women's Training College to attend just one clinic, as their campuses were adjacent. This again saved me time later on when there were more demands on it.

Equipment was of the most basic. In each place I was provided with a bed to act as an examination couch – generally with just a sleeping mat on instead of a mattress (except for the girls' establishments). I always had a table and a chair, so that I had somewhere to put my records while I wrote them up. I carried all records with me – none were ever left in the schools. I tried to give as much treatment on the spot as I could, which meant that injections were often needed – penicillin for infections, and other injections for ailments such as bilharzia, from which many of the pupils and students

200

suffered, particularly when they returned from their villages at the end of the vacations.

The dispensary attendant at the Craft School had one or two syringes, but I can't imagine what his needles were like – no needles were ever sharpened – we had no facilities for sophisticated procedures like that. I had my own set of syringes though, and a small portable steriliser into which they fitted. Each time I went home on leave I had replenished my supply of needles, and I never let anyone else use any of them in Nigeria, for I needed to look after them myself and husband them – they all had to last for at least a year. I was able to ensure, therefore, that even injection treatment could be given within the schools and colleges.

In addition to that side of the service, I decided that I would examine each pupil or student every term, as soon after they returned from holidays as possible. As I have just said, many would come back with signs of bilharzia. Others would have become anaemic, perhaps because of malaria, maybe because of parasites like hookworm. Many would have ringworm, or scabies, or other skin problems. Yet others would have eye infections. They all, I felt needed to be sorted out as soon as possible and treated, so that they could benefit more from their teaching. I also examined every newcomer at the start of each academic year. It was amazing what turned up. I can remember one small boy who came to the Secondary School as a new pupil. Only the brightest children went there, as they would sit for the West African School Certificate and several would hope to go to university eventually. So this child must have shown promise. He was really small compared with the others, and no wonder, because when I checked him I found that he was on the verge of cardiac failure due to a congenital abnormality of his heart. He must indeed have been very bright to have made it to this school. I was pleased to note over the following months how much his general condition improved when he was having a really well organised day and a good balanced diet. All in all, the school service for which I had agreed to be employed for only half-time, began to take up more and more hours as the weeks went on.

I had said I would do and be paid for no more than half-time so that with a clear conscience I could take time at home should any crisis occur within my family, and even later on when I found that I was once again working round the clock I didn't change that arrangement. And there were a few times when I was glad of it too, when there was illness at home and I could be around there. Nevertheless, I managed to do two sessions weekly at each school and the two colleges.

I have mentioned my records. I had to devise these myself. There was no precedent for any of this, there having never been any school service before. I bought exercise books from the mission bookshop, and ruled them out into a format which enabled me not only record the daily clinic work and treatment, but also the regular medical examinations. I had no resources allowed for that, so did it all myself. It took hours of time getting the books ready, but it was time well spent, and I was able to send regular full reports to Kaduna of what I had been doing. For request slips to the lab, and prescriptions I had to use any scraps of paper that I could come by. I had no proper request forms, so that I tore bits of paper that remained blank from bigger sheets which had been used for something else. But what I did served perfectly well. No wonder none of us ever threw anything away – everything could be made use of somehow, and my little school service was no exception. I hoped that the powers that be would see what a boon this service was and that one day they might perhaps factor it in as part of the general Education system.

After several months of doing this, and finding that it seemed to be successful, I decided to try to extend it in a simple way to the Native Authority schools in the town. In all there were ten of these as well as two Mission schools – one Anglican and one Roman Catholic. There was one dispensary attendant in the town who did what he could in the way of treating schoolchildren, but now I was able to give him a good deal of help and guidance, as well as doing regular medical inspections for all those children too. The days became very full!

In March 1962 we had a second child. He was born at the Maiduguri Nursing Home, which had finally been opened regularly, as for the time being, there were now enough staff to run it. Once again I had been fit enough not to be sent elsewhere for the birth, and also, luckily for me, one of the two medical officers in Maiduguri at the time had an obstetric qualification. I knew I was in good hands. Our son was born as dawn came at the end of the last night of Ramadan. There was always competition between Maiduguri and Sokoto at this time, each wanting to be the first to see the new moon and to announce the end of Ramadan. Whether or not Maiduguri was the first this time I don't know – but just as my son was delivered the cannons went off to signal the end of the fast. That being so, all the Africans promptly called him 'Alhaji', telling us that any boy baby born on that day was always given that name. And Alhaji he remained for many of them as long as we stayed in Nigeria. It seemed somehow right that our children had both been born in Nigeria, and it was strange to think that they had both been born on special days – one on Christmas Eve, a Christian festival, and the other at the end of Ramadan, an Islamic festival day.

For the first months of his life I didn't work, not until he was bigger. But when I did start again, I knew that it would not be feasible to try to take two children around with me, and we engaged a child minder. Our reliable and 'very decent' Mr Ita produced Grace, who came from his tribe and who he knew well. She was a jolly woman, plump and comfortable and the children loved her from the start. We knew that Mr Ita would not have recommended her unless she was really all right, and I had no qualms about leaving our two with her. I always got them up myself each day before going to work, and I was always home again to see to their meals myself. Often I nipped home in the middle of the morning as well, just to reassure myself that everything was all right. Grace would arrive at about eight o'clock each morning, and she looked after the children until lunch time when I took over. After lunch they would sleep and I would too, and Grace watched out for them during siesta until I surfaced, after which she would go home. Although she always walked to work, I often gave her a lift back into town, which she and the children enjoyed.

As time went on, I was asked to take on more duties. Now that the nursing home was permanently open for both out-and in-patients, I was detailed off to look after it totally, and from time to time I was asked to look on at the hospital as well.

Life really was busy, and there were occasions now when I would put the children to bed at the end of the day, go to the nursing home for some emergency and only just get back home in time to get them up again in the morning. Luckily Rex was always at home to be there for them if I was called out. Without his willing help I don't know how I would have managed. I was effectively working full time plus.

It wasn't all work of course – we still managed to have a social life, having friends in for meals, offering hospitality to various guests and even managing to have an occasional evening out, if a friend would come and babysit for us. As the wife of the college Principal, I was also expected to involve myself with college affairs to some extent. I judged various competitions, watched 'official' football matches as well as being responsible for hospitality to and entertaining of, various VIP guests. One occasion which demanded my attendance, was the Maiduguri 'Independence Football Match' for which Rex had been asked to be the referee, to his delight. He had been both a good footballer and an excellent sprinter when younger, though he now confined himself to playing tennis. However, he was more than capable of running up and down the pitch blowing a whistle. Members of the hospital staff made up one of the two teams, and I well remember one of our nurses, Paul Okafor, taking part. My husband always said what a good footballer Paul was. He was an excellent nurse too, conscientious and intelligent. We were told some years later that he was killed in the first big uprising before the civil war. A waste of a young life.

We continued to have unexpected visitors. Before we were engaged, a man had walked in one day to the P.E.O's office, in Maiduguri, introducing himself as Professor Lukas, Professor of African languages at Hamburg University. Rex almost said to this dusty, travel stained and unexpected stranger, "Oh yes, and I'm the Queen of Sheba," but luckily didn't, for his visitor was indeed who he said he was. Prof Lukas spent a lot of his long vacations in going to different African countries, in order to learn yet more tribal languages. He was in Maiduguri for several weeks, and the rest of the station made sure that he too was included in the speculation about whether or not Rex and I would become engaged at the next party either of us hosted. Some years later on when we were back in Maiduguri, he returned, bringing his wife with him as he had done before. This time they found us well married and with a young family. It was good to see them again.

In Katsina once we had been surprised to see a Land Rover drive into our compound, out of which climbed several dusty and rather tired young men. They were medical students who had spent much of their long vacation driving across the Sahara, doing all sorts of physiological experiments on themselves en route. They had just come in off the desert, and had found their way to the hospital to ask for the medical officer. They were more than glad of the pints of half frozen lager from our fridge that we poured down their throats before they went on to the Rest House. Shades of 'Ice Cold in Alex'!

Another unexpected arrival, again hot and dusty from the road, was the State Librarian from Western Australia, who was on a sabbatical and who also had his wife with him. They had driven up from Jos, I think, and said that they saw the sign to the college and simply drove up to try to find somebody who could tell them where the Rest House was. Why Maiduguri had been in his sights I don't know. Perhaps he was interested in schools and colleges. We certainly had a good library at our college.

I cannot now recall everyone who visited, but I remember one man who later became President of Nigeria, some years after Independence. There was a day when Rex came down from the college accompanied by a smart young army officer. It seemed that army manoeuvres were to be held in and around Maiduguri. The young man had approached my husband to ask if the soldiers might use the college playing fields now and again while they were in the area. He sat and chatted to us over drinks for a little while before getting back to base. We had the soldiers sharing the football pitch with the students for a week or two. Years later, when General Gowon became President and his photograph was in the national newspapers, we looked at one another and said, "That looks like our young army officer." Like I said, you never knew who would turn up. Life was nothing if not interesting in Nigeria.

Rex had now met two people who were to become Presidents of Nigeria. The first was Mallam Shehu Shigari, who was, at the time Rex knew him, a teacher. He was, some time after they had first met, sent to the UK to do a course there. My husband had not been on leave then, but had given Shehu Shigari his parents' address and asked him to contact them. They promptly invited this young Nigerian to stay with them for a few days, which he did. My in-laws had both died shortly after our marriage, and Rex often said to me, "Wouldn't my parents have been interested to know how their guest of so many years before had ended up?"

As well as running a school medical service locally, I would have liked to extend it to nearby bush schools. However, from 1962 onwards, with two infants of my own to look after, that clearly was not possible – I had to accept that my touring days were over. Still, I did manage to visit one or two outlying schools that were not too far away, and examined the children there, and tried to sort out some minor ailments there as well. It was interesting to note that before I laid a hand on a child at all, the teachers at every school I went to said, ostensibly to show the children that a medical examination was quite harmless, "Watch me, then you'll see what happens" and then whipped off their caftans or *rigas* and presented themselves as the first to be examined. I think the *Mallams* (the teachers) were eager to be checked over themselves, and were not going to miss out on such an opportunity. Well, the more the merrier. They had as little chance as the children to be seen unless they managed to get to Maiduguri in school holidays.

What I did succeed in organising, though, in March 1963, was for teachers from bush schools to come to Maiduguri during one or two of the shorter breaks between terms in order to attend a simple first aid course, together with an equally simple course that I devised for them on treatment of minor conditions. I also, by dint of twisting a few arms at the hospital, put together a small supply of first aid kit and aspirins for them to use at school. I suspect that some of the supplies would be used up, or even sold on, very soon after they returned to school, but it was a start and they seemed to enjoy the short training period and I hope I sowed a few seeds of knowledge there.

One of the best things that happened for the schools, which turned up right out of the blue in August 1963, was that a Health Sister came to give BCG vaccinations to pupils and students. The vaccinations were preceded by skin testing. Vaccinations were only given to those whose skin tests were negative. I still have the reports on the numbers of children seen, tested and vaccinated in respect of a couple of the town schools. The teachers there were also tested. I welcomed this development, for there was so much tuberculosis around, often of the severity of cases I had treated in England before we had streptomycin and other drugs available. It was interesting to note in one Junior Primary School, that two thirds of the children were not vaccinated as they already had positive skin tests. In another school, a Senior Primary, where the children were a year or two older, just over three quarters of the children had positive skin tests and only a few were therefore vaccinated. I wonder if this scheme was continued after the civil war. I hope so. There was so much TB among the general population, and as it was known to be infectious, people would not easily admit to illness, feeling that there was a stigma attached to it. They seemed to be far more willing to come for advice about leprosy, which surprised me, when I thought of how lepers have been feared and driven away from society throughout history. Perhaps because there were specific leprosy hospitals, people felt more secure about it, whereas at the time I was in Nigeria, I had not come across sanatoria for tuberculous patients.

Chapter 23

I think at this point I should say something about the Bornu Men's Teacher Training College. I have mentioned it and my husband often during this memoir, but have not really gone into any detail.

I feel it worth taking some time over, because it was a big undertaking, and probably something not really experienced here in the UK in the same way. In Britain there would probably be a series of committees, all dealing with different arrangements when starting off a training college. A librarian would be appointed to order and catalogue recommended books. A dietician would organise food supplies and menus. Tutors and heads of departments would work out syllabuses and timetables.

Here in Maiduguri one man had to undertake everything himself, and with the first class of students but no other member of teaching staff, he also had to teach for every lesson in the week. It took a great deal of organisation. But every education officer in Nigeria, as I have already probably indicated, had to be prepared to take on any sort of job anywhere in the country. Rex had already done wide administrative duties as Provincial Education Officer, which was a job like a sort of local Director of Education, dealing with all the administration and school inspections in a province. He had taught at a boys' secondary school in Kano; he had run an outlying branch of a men's teacher training college in yet another province; he had been second in command at the Katsina Training College, and now he was to be the Principal of the new Bornu Men's Teacher Training College.

He had, as has been said, taken over the first class of students, then housed temporarily in a small mud building, later transferring them to much better accommodation but not yet to the custom-built premises which were still under construction. Eventually the new college campus was completed and the buildings formally handed over to the Principal. The college buildings comprised not only those directly concerned with the students, but also the staff houses for both senior service and junior staff, so that the Principal needed to know if there were any problems there at any time, though so far as structural problems were concerned he would refer to the local Public Works Department.

At this point the really hard work began, for much had to be provided and arranged before a single student could move in.

The students all had to be housed and fed for starters. So in advance of the move, the Principal had to invite tenders for the supply of things like tables and chairs, beds, mosquito nets, and eating utensils. He had to invite applications for cooks, and labourers – all daily paid staff. He had to work out diets and meals which would be well balanced and nutritious for everyone, while at the same time being acceptable for several different tribes and religions. And he had to invite tenders for the supply of food materials from various contractors in the town.

He had to design a college uniform, with different outfits for different occasions. There was to be a 'walking out' uniform to be worn if students went off-campus, for example into town for any reason. There was another uniform for everyday classroom wear. The Principal had to choose colours for and design both outfits. He had to find and engage tailors who would come to the college and measure all the students for their uniforms, before making the clothes and delivering them back to the college. He had to source and purchase the fabrics to be used. He also had to select and order games strips and PE kit, together with equipment for various sports – football, hockey, volleyball and so on.

Between us we designed a crest for the college badge. Rex decided that the college colours would be blue and white, and asked me to draw and colour a representation of what he wanted. This I did as well as I could, using the old watercolour paint-box that I'd kept ever since my schooldays (and which I still have, together with that original effort). In his handing over notes Rex gave the following description:

'The badge is in the form of a shield, its heraldic description being 'Azure, in chief a Northern Knot between two open books, in base three crown birds volant one over one all argent.' You will see the badge on the signboards at the bottom of the main drive.'

To engender a sense of pride in the college and also to ensure that the students all vied with one another in their attempts to keep the whole college a flagship institution, he set up a House system. Every student on admission was allocated to one of three Houses, each of which had been given a name of a past ruler of Bornu: Kyari, El Kanemi and Aloma.

There was the question of whether the college should have any kind of regular general assembly each week, and if so what form should it take? There would be students from more than one religion – could they have a religious assembly or should it be simply a sort of business meeting?

There were other questions that occurred to him as well. How would he know, for instance, if the students kept the college really clean and tidy or if they let everything drift into scenes of chaos, both in the classrooms and in the dormitories? How would he know if they did their academic tasks, wrote

208

their essays and so on? Would he be getting any new lecturers at all and what would their special subjects be?

There was a library to equip – students without reference books would be handicapped from the start. And there was no games field, just a large area of virgin bush where it should be. Taylor Woodrow had not been asked to make football pitches or anything like that.

Gradually things began to happen. Tailors came with all sorts of patterns, colours and materials, measured up the students and sent in their estimates. Local women from different tribes turned up offering their services as cooks, and were presented with a sample menu to see if they thought they could produce it regularly, the menu having been put together after consultation with several people from the tribes and religions first. Labourers and night watchmen were appointed, as well as, importantly, a college Sergeant. He was an ex-soldier who saw to the college timekeeping, and supervised the staff under him – cooks, labourers and so on.

Rex decided that he would follow a method of weekly inspections of kit and surroundings that he had been accustomed to when in the Navy during World War 2. Once a week, he would go round the dormitories accompanied by a member of staff and the senior student. Here each student had to lay out his college-provided uniforms and other kit on his bed, and the rooms had to be cleanly swept, as had the classrooms. We did not have domestic staff to do these tasks and the students themselves were responsible for all that. One important thing to check on inspection days was the condition of all the mosquito nets. The impression that we had was that nets were often considered to be a bit of a status symbol. Students would probably not have them at home in their villages. It was quite something, therefore, to have a net for your bed. However, should the net get torn, people did not bother to mend it – it was enough just to have a net. It didn't seem to matter that the value of a net lay in its wholeness and not in its 'hole-iness', and the students had to be told to mend their nets as and when necessary.

After consultation with the local Imam and a member of the Christian Mission, with the use of books of both Moslem and Christian prayers, a format was arrived at for a weekly college assembly. In the first week the Principal would give a Moslem reading and a Christian prayer, which were acceptable to both religions, and the following week he would give a Christian reading and a Moslem prayer, and so on for alternate weeks throughout the college terms. These were taken from a Book of Prayers and Readings approved also by the College Advisory Board. Everyone was happy about that, and it was felt that the right note had been struck. It went down well with all the students and there was never any discord over it. After these readings, Rex would give out any notices before the students went into class. It was felt that this weekly assembly would enable students to feel that they belonged to a 'whole', rather than separate units, and would bind them together.

The games fields posed a bit of a problem at first, as no money was allocated for hacking these out of bush. However, by dint of asking round various departments, Rex managed to beg the use of a tractor/grader from an American Aid project that was concerned with building a cattle ranch just outside Maiduguri. Two of his teaching staff volunteered to have a go at operating it in order to level the necessary areas for football and hockey pitches, and areas for volleyball and other minor games. He solved the problem of goal posts by using old unwanted lengths of scaffolding from the PWD. Nets he had to buy from petty cash, so far as I recall.

The last big job which the Principal had to face – and this he had to do personally and regularly, was to pay the students. All students were given an allocation of pocket money at regular intervals, and they were also paid a sum of money for their travelling costs at the beginning and end of each term. Incidentally, all their journeys to and from their homes had to be organised by the Principal in time for the relevant dates, so that there could be no excuses for late or non-arrivals. Payday was a very long day, for nobody ever wanted to be paid in anything but coinage, which meant that Rex and his clerk spent hours of time setting out piles of shillings on a table before having the students lined up by the college sergeant, then to come one by one to receive and sign for their money. This was counted out in front of each one, coin by coin so that nobody would be accused of cheating them. It wasn't so bad when there was just the one class to pay, but as the college grew, the task became very arduous indeed and took whole days to complete. Still, it had to be done.

One very enjoyable task which my husband tackled, having got the most practical matters sorted out to his satisfaction before we went on leave prior to moving into the new college, was to give thought to the stocking up of a library. The college had a lovely big library building, with many shelves, but as yet no books. He began to put a list together in good time, adding to it as he thought of what might be needed, and when we went on leave we spent a wonderful afternoon at a big bookshop back in the UK, ordering all the books he had listed. On first going into the shop, and saying that he wanted to 'buy some books', the assistant seemed not to take him all that seriously, clearly thinking that here was some nutcase who just wanted a few yards of books – any books – on his shelves. Gradually he realised that Rex had several hundred pounds to spend, and that he was starting up a real college library from scratch, and his attitude changed remarkably. We smiled at this afterwards. Several hundred pounds was a lot of money then – nothing like so much now. That afternoon was fun for us both, and it left a great feeling of satisfaction – which was even greater when the crates arrived in Nigeria at the appointed time and were unpacked and the books stacked on the shelves. At first, although we had spent so much money on books, they looked more than sparse when we first put them up on the shelves, but as time went on, the gaps were gradually filled, and before we retired, the library was something to be quite proud of.

The students all settled in to the new premises and I am sure much appreciated them, as indeed we did. The labourers began to clear the spaces between buildings and planted shrubs and flowers there, so that the whole place soon began to look very attractive. When we saw that weaver birds were beginning to build their nests around the campus, we felt that it had really got itself established. The Rural Science tutor (who was always an African) got the students to clear another area of bush on to which they then set out a series of small 'gardens' so that each could have his own patch to cultivate. This area also soon began to look well ordered, and each day at the end of the afternoon, while it was still light, the students turned out willingly to tend their various plots. However, not all the students worked on their gardens on the same days. The end of the afternoons between 4 p.m. and about 5.30 p.m. was the time allocated for games as well, so that those who were down to play games did their gardening on other days, while the gardeners on one day would find themselves down for games on another. The games were very popular with everybody, as were also athletics. We were lucky to have two tutors who specialised in PE and games. One was a young Englishman, Laurie Parker – in fact the first member of staff to be appointed after Rex took over the college. Another was a member of the US Peace Corps, a very fit young chap. I can remember him taking a bunch of students on a cross country run, and when they were coming back up the road on the home run and all looking extremely tired, he was there in front of them, encouraging them on and getting them home – and he was running backwards! He didn't seem to be the slightest bit weary, and was watching them and willing them on. Nobody dropped out of line.

I have said that the Rural Science tutors were always Nigerian. The Arabist was also a Nigerian, a nice man, quiet and efficient. He taught Religious Education (Islamic) to the Moslem students, and oversaw their pastoral care. One of the expatriates at the Christian Mission taught R.E. to the Christian students and oversaw their welfare, though my husband made a point of knowing all his students personally as well – as far as was possible in a growing college.

Before long we had another Nigerian tutor posted to the college who taught Art, and who started off what became a flourishing Art Club. My husband encouraged as many clubs and societies at the college as people

211

could cope with. He also started off a college magazine, for not only did these things provide interest within the college, but also they gave the students ideas about what they might organise within the schools where they would eventually teach, at least he hoped that might happen. In fact, it would probably be a very long time before such things could be arranged in some of the bush schools, for the communities in outlying districts could be poor, and the children would be expected to work and not 'play' if they were not actually attending lessons. It was not easy introducing new ideas to far away villages. Having found so much bilharzia among school children and students returning from holidays, I tried, in the hygiene lessons I gave, to teach the older ones how to guard against bilharzia. But the next term they would arrive back with re-infections. "We told our families what you had said," they would tell me, "but they just said that it might be all right to do these things at college, but they were not what we did in our villages. Now we were at home we must do what had always been done in the village and not bring newfangled ideas home with us."

When I re-read the comprehensive handing-over notes that Rex gave to the incoming Principal when we finally retired from service in Nigeria, I am still amazed at the innumerable details which he outlined, and which were all part of the organisation that he had visualised and set up himself from scratch.

After the college had been running smoothly in its new campus for some time, and therefore after everything had been properly organised, games fields, gardens, teaching schedules and so on, Rex decided in early 1962 that it would be nice to have an official opening ceremony. As far as I recall this would have been late January or early February because it was still Harmattan then and the roads remained passable for those coming from a distance.

He first of all invited the Sardauna of Sokoto, Sir Amadu Bello, to perform the opening. Yes, he was told, the Sardauna would be delighted to come. Then he invited the local Native Authority officials, all of whom accepted. The Minister for Education, Alhaji Isa Kaita said that he would attend. The Provincial Commissioner for Bornu, an African official appointed since Independence to replace the British Resident, and who now lived in what had been the Residency, said he would come. Rex also discovered that for some reason which I now forget, the President of French Niger was coming to Maiduguri on a sort of state visit just at that time, so extended an invitation to him as well, that being simple courtesy. Yes, he would be pleased to attend, together with his entourage. And the Waziri of Bornu, Shettima Kashim Ibrahim would also be there. It was to be quite an event.

Everything was cleaned, polished and arranged for the big day. The students made sure that their walking-out uniforms were in good order and that the dormitories and classrooms were spick and span for people to visit.

Rex decided that it might be a diplomatic gesture not only to fly the Nigerian flag for the occasion, but also the flag of Niger since that country's President was coming. So he got one of the tailors in the town to run up the two flags. The obvious place to hoist them was, he thought, at the entrance to the long drive as it opened off the main airport road. But he had no flag poles. A hasty inquiry to the Public Works Department solved the problem and he was told that they would make two flagpoles out of scaffolding. They could be carried down to the end of the drive for the occasion, and then returned to PWD for dismantling afterwards. Fine. That solved the problem beautifully.

In due course the flagpoles arrived at the college – the scaffolding had been used to make a square base and a fitment for vertical poles to be fixed in, with ropes attached so that flags could be run up. It was a perfectly satisfactory construction, but rather heavy and would need several men to carry each one to its appointed place. Because of possible theft, they were kept at the college until the morning of the Opening day. When it was time to manhandle them down the long drive, the labourers were detailed off accordingly, three or four men to each, and off they went, carrying these heavy and rather awkward devices. A few minutes later on, when they were expected back at the college to say that whoever was to hoist the flags could now go along and get on with it, a man came sprinting up the drive alone, in a total panic.

'Dead men everywhere!' was all he could say. He seemed very shocked. When anyone could get any sense out of him, he said that on the way down the drive, those carrying the flagpoles suddenly all collapsed and fell to the ground, and lost consciousness.

Several members of staff rushed along, to find that this was indeed so. Nobody, neither senior nor junior staff had realised that some power lines crossed the college drive, obscured by overhanging tree branches and in any case were not very high. The labourers who carried the flagpoles had simply picked them up by their bases so that the poles were carried vertically, rather than distributing the weight more evenly by carrying them horizontally. It had been only too easy for the tops of the metal poles to hit the power lines. I was called and ran down from our house, sending for students who had done the first aid course that I had taught, to find bodies lying across the drive just as they had fallen. Most seemed dead but nevertheless the students and I set to work on artificial respiration while somebody phoned the hospital and asked for the ambulance to be sent forthwith. Heavily pregnant I just hoped I would not go into early labour as I helped to heave the men into the ambulance and continued artificial respiration until we reached the hospital. Everyone was very subdued after this – a terrible way to embark on what was intended to be a special day in the history of the college. However the show had to go on. The important visitors and heads of departments, native authority officials and students were due to take their places in another hour or two. So in spite of the morning's horrific tragedy, everyone pulled together to in order to ensure that the college opening was enjoyed by all the visitors.

The Africans were resplendent in their robes and colourful head coverings, *hulas*, turbans and so on. The Minister for Saharan Affairs from Niger wore a spotlessly white veil as well, in true Tuareg style. The Sardauna of Sokoto had a purple velvet robe with lots of gold embroidery on it – a beautiful garment and very impressive. All the expatriate Government heads of departments attended too. It was a well received event altogether, and something for the college to remember.

I kept myself out of the way most of the time, and slunk about as invisibly as I could, trying to take photographs unobtrusively, sometimes bumping into the official press cameraman, who was a bit dismissive of all the fuss. He said, when trying to get a shot of the Sardauna, "Catch him just going in through a door, and then catch him coming out again, that's all." He'd seen it all before!

The speeches made, all the college buildings and departments inspected, hands shaken and greetings exchanged, the important visitors returned to their limousines and drove off. Rex thankfully took off his hot academic gown (a good foil to all the African robes, I think), and changed his suit and tie for more comfortable shorts and thin shirt, and relaxed for the rest of the day. It had been hard work, but well worth it. Ceremony was understood and appreciated, and gave a value to things. In this newly independent Nigeria, education was going to be important. The Bornu Men's Teacher Training College was new, well organised, it was already growing and many families already wanted their sons to attend there, and I like to think it was a bit of a flagship at that time.

When it was time for the Principal to recruit for the next academic year, he was frequently offered large sums of money to accept this or that boy. Fathers who had some wealth would come in person long before the recommendations had arrived from the schools, waving wads of notes in front of him to tempt him to say that he would take in their sons. His reply was always the same: "Your son, if he applies, will be seen by me at interview, and I will also receive a report of his school work from his headmaster. That is when I will decide if he will or will not be accepted here. I do not take payments for accepting students. That is not what we do. They are admitted to college on their personal suitability for the training offered here."

There might have been disappointment at what he said, but there was never any offence taken. There might also have been some puzzlement, for the payment of money for favours was one of the ways of life in Nigeria.

Chapter 24

I can't let this memoir go without some mention of elections. I remember two big elections being held. Because of the possibility of trouble outside the polling stations, or cheating over the counting of votes, or both, the Europeans always seemed to be sent to supervise in some capacity.

When we were in Katsina, my husband was sent once to a place called Funtua, a small township 140 miles from Katsina, to preside over the actual ballot, and also to act as returning officer for when the ballot was counted. He was warned that there was great rivalry, not always friendly, between the two opposing parties there, and trouble was considered to be more than likely. The polling station, therefore, was under military armed guard. Luckily the popular party won, so that no fighting broke out and he came back home with nothing worse in the way of trauma than several huge blisters on his hands – the result of trying to turn the keys in the ballot box locks – they were almost corroded in, and everyone there had in turn struggled before the boxes were finally opened

This was, in fact, a pretty exhausting week for Rex (the first week in December 1959), for on the Thursday he drove me to Kano where I would stay until the birth of our baby, and he returned to Katsina the same day – 200 miles of bumpy road in all. The next day he went to Funtua, over a bush road, in preparation for the election on the Saturday. After supervising the voting all day long while the polling station was open, he had to be awake and alert for the count, which started at 7 pm on polling day and continued until 4 pm the next day, Sunday. On the Monday he had to drive another 100 miles to Kaduna for a conference, and the day after that he drove from Kaduna to Kano to see me before returning to Katsina where at last he could have a good sleep. In the end we stopped counting the hundreds of miles he had driven during that week! At least it wasn't the rainy season, so that the roads, even if rough, were dry

The other election was held when we were back in Maiduguri. Rex was told that he had to go east to Potiskum, about 160 miles along the road to Jos, to act once again as presiding officer and to supervise the voting and the count afterwards, following which he had to announce the result. Because most people could neither read nor write, the ballot papers couldn't have candidates' names written on them. Instead, the various parties were indicated by pictures of different animals, and everyone knew which animal represented which party. So people simply put a thumbprint or a cross next

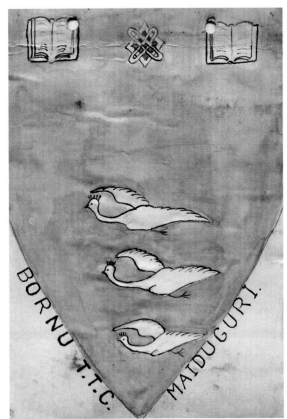

The rough and ready original design and colours for the Bornu Men's Teacher Training College crest, which I drew and painted to Rex's specifications.

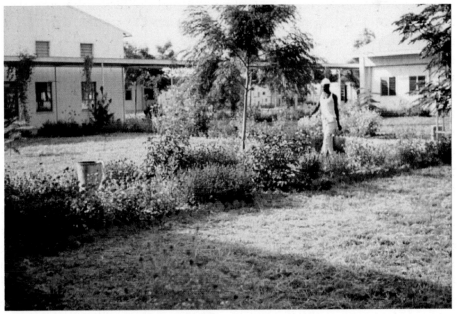

The Bornu Teacher Training College gardens become well-established. 'Administration Rose' (Portulaca) in the foreground.

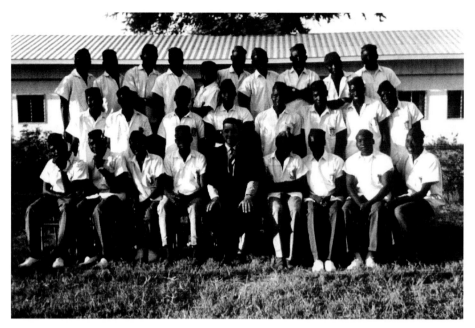

Rex Abraham (Principal) and the senior students at Bornu Training
College, 1964.

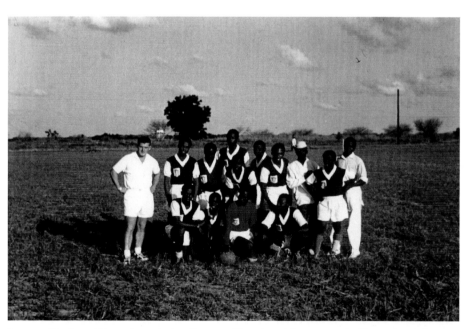

Laurie Parker (Tutor) and the Bornu Teacher Training College 1st XI
football team, wearing the blue and white college colours.

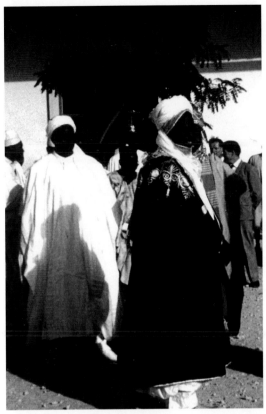

Alhaji Sir Ahmadu Bello, Sardauna of Sokoto, Premier of Northern Nigeria (in dark robe), officially opens the Bornu Men's Teacher Training College in 1962.

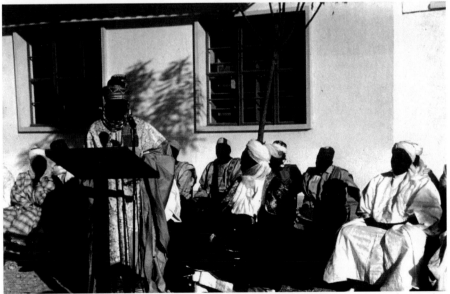

Alhaji Isa Kaita, Minister for Education, Northern Nigeria, speaks at the official opening of Bornu Men's Teacher Training College, 1962.

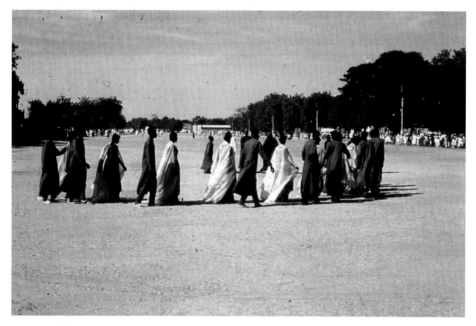

Kanuri dancers on the Dandal Way, Maiduguri, entertain the crowds after a durbar has ended, c. 1960.

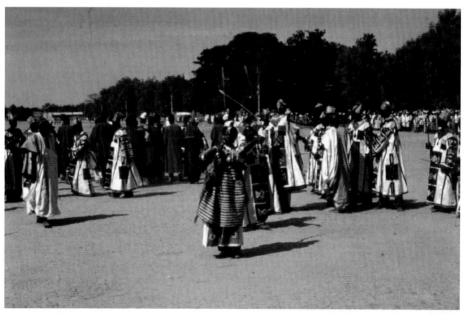

More dancers at the Maiduguri durbar.

to whichever animal they favoured. It was, said my husband, a long day and an even longer night, but finally the voting finished, and he then presided over the count. Again it was a popular result and people were very happy about it.

Rex's own car was waiting for new tyres so that he dare not risk it on the long journey to Potiskum. That being the case, he borrowed mine for the trip. The day after the election, therefore, I looked for my Opel to come trundling up the drive, and was surprised to see a Land Rover stop outside the house. When Rex got out of that I was even more surprised. "Before you ask," he said, "Your car has been rather badly damaged, and as I am carrying the ballot boxes, I have managed to borrow this Land Rover because it was sure to get here safely. I shall be taken back to Potiskum tomorrow to collect your car, which is still just about driveable, luckily."

My car was rather badly damaged? What on earth had happened? What had happened was as follows.

Rex, having completed the count and announced the result, had loaded up my car and set off from the polling station, which was on a side road. Ahead of him were vast crowds, all rejoicing and celebrating. Slowly he inched through the mass of people on his way to the main road to Maiduguri. Suddenly the crowds fell away, leaving a huge clear space in front and on either side of him, along which he realised, to his consternation, that three horsemen were galloping full pelt in a sort of miniature durbar, spears and swords waving as they approached, and all of them yelling in celebration. There was no time to do anything, the crowd was pressing against him from in front and behind, and the horsemen were coming from the side. As they crashed into the car, a spear went through the passenger door, just missing the man travelling with him, and one of the horses tried to jump over the vehicle, its hooves landing on the roof as it did so. The passenger side of the car was totally written off, there was a great hole through the door, the door itself hung from its hinges, and there were huge dents and scrapes on the roof. Luckily the car, as he said, was still just driveable, and the next day he brought it back to Maiduguri.

I arranged for repairs to be done, and sent a claim in to the insurers. I was not best pleased when the insurers wrote to me to say that no payment would be forthcoming. "Had it been a riot," they told me, "we would have paid because that would have been covered. But this was not a riot, it was rejoicing and happiness, and that doesn't count. Sorry."

Car insurance was quite heavy in Nigeria because of the frequency of accidents with African drivers on the roads, even though there was nothing like the traffic there (except for the traffic in the big towns and cities, where it could be horrendous, with every rule of the road in the book being broken all the time).

Elections remind me (don't ask me why!) of a time when a population census was organised. Official census recorders were appointed, and travelled round the country, into the towns and out into bush villages and other habitations. In due course the returns were scrutinised. It was then discovered that (in Bornu at least, and very likely elsewhere for all I know) a method of counting heads had been used which was not exactly expected. It was found, we were told, that if the recorder visited a household in which somebody had recently died but the body had not yet been moved, then that person was counted, as they considered that he or she was still there. Similarly, if a visit was made to a house where a baby was imminently to be born, then the baby was counted on the census because it was so nearly there in its own right.

Another count had to be organised. This time, a large contingent of ladies from Lagos was sent up to Bornu. They arrived, more than a little disgruntled with their mode of transport which was a large Mammy wagon that had bumped and jolted them all the way from the big city. I especially remember seeing them arrive – they all had brightly coloured umbrellas to use as parasols. I heard afterwards that they complained bitterly about this posting, for they thought that Bornu was the most 'bush' place they had seen and they had not been best pleased with the accommodation arranged for them. Ah, the sophistication of Lagos! I expect they were all glad to return to its creature comforts.

As the Bornu College grew, the existing dormitory accommodation was no longer enough for all the students to be able to board. Arrangements had to be made therefore for some to live in digs in the town. This was never satisfactory while we were there, partly because the local population was not geared to the idea of anyone settling down in the evenings to write essays or do any reading or revision. There was always too much noise – and too many temptations to join in whatever fun was going on anyway. There were also health implications to having students living out.

One day it was reported to me that one of the students had been caught by the police for smoking cannabis (Indian Hemp, as it was then called). This was something that to our knowledge had not happened before, and was a worrying development. I knew already that there was some drug taking in town, but until then I don't think there had been very much, unless you considered 'iska' – the 'spirits' – in the form of some local brew which the locals occasionally ate or drank, to be 'drugs'. Now the drug scene as we know it had come to Maiduguri, albeit, as yet, in a small way.

Another health bombshell which fell, once students had to live in the town was that I began to see cases of venereal disease in the school and college clinics – among the students and schoolboys, that is, and not among the girls who always had to be chaperoned carefully if they ever went to the town for anything. In the first years of the college when there were only one or two classes, and after my Health and Hygiene teaching which included instruction about VD, we had not had any cases at all. Once the college grew, the odd case appeared. Now, with students actually living in the town, the occasional case multiplied. I had no idea how to prevent this from happening other than to reinforce what I taught. I no longer did any classroom teaching for I simply didn't have time, but I said what I could in my clinics and hoped that something might sink in to the minds of a few people. I knew how rife venereal disease was in the town, and what devastating effects it could and did have.

It was interesting to me, as I am back now with the school clinics for a moment, to see how the attitude of some of the children and students towards illness altered after they had been with us for a short time. On admission to school or college, as I have said, I tried to do an initial medical examination for each new entrant. Some were in a very poor state of health really when they arrived – perhaps anaemic, with skin rashes, maybe parasites, hookworm, tapeworm, scabies, whatever, but generally below par. Some must have felt quite out of sorts really. They were quite stoical about their various ailments, their general attitude being 'everybody had something wrong with them didn't they?' They just put up with any discomfort.

But after a few weeks all this changed. I began to realise that some were turning up at the clinics demanding treatment for the most trivial of complaints – things that I myself would never have dreamed of seeking advice for, even if I were a laywoman. Now they were insisting that I gave medicine, injections, sick notes, sent them to hospital, and they could be quite put out when I told them that there was no special treatment, say, for a cold apart from the odd aspirin. Eventually the message got through and my clinics returned to normality except for a small hard core of those who always tried it on. But that happens everywhere – it is human nature.

I haven't mentioned eye troubles. I did not do any eye testing for I had no equipment with which to do any. However at one time we had an Egyptian eye specialist as the MO in charge at the Maiduguri General Hospital. He was a nice man who, in spite of his being a specialist, didn't mind rolling up his sleeves and having a go at anything else if help was needed. I often sent children to him for eye problems that I could not deal with myself. Otherwise if there was any great problem, the nearest place was Kano, 400 miles away. To get there was expensive, but even so, an occasional patient managed to make the journey. Others had to put up with their short sight or other problems. Trachoma and conjunctivitis and simple complaints of that sort could be dealt with by us in Maiduguri, and there were plenty of such cases around all the time. We would see a lot of conjunctivitis during the Harmattan because of all the stinging dust.

There was also a good deal of blindness among the adults due to long standing trachoma as well as because of cataracts. Blind people would manage to get about because they all seemed to have a child on hand who would lead them around. The sufferer would hold the end of a long stick and the child would hold the other end and would walk in front, so that the blind man or woman behind would simply go where the stick pulled. It seemed to work well, and what was given to them (for they often begged) would buy a little food. There was a so-called 'Blind School' in Maiduguri – for adults, but only a few people seemed to go there. I never discovered how it was financed, perhaps the Native Authority backed it. There they would weave mats, some for sleeping, while others would be big enough to cover floors. They would make other small goods too. Some of the woven work was always displayed at the local Agricultural Show.

Have I described the Agricultural Show in Maiduguri yet? It was one of our 'big' annual events, and always enjoyable. Mallam Lawan was the Provincial Agricultural Officer, and he, along with the then expatriate Agricultural Officer would organise it. A large arena was used, and here many animals would be shown - sheep, cattle, horses, camels. The animals would be paraded round the show ring with pride. At one end examples of the local crops would be on display - corn several feet high, for instance, which I found to be very impressive. In the rainy season, you could just about see it growing, I always thought. There would be a small gymkhana too, with fairly low jumps, over which local riders would compete on their best horses. That was always fun to watch. In the middle of the area there would usually be displayed one or two small huts made from *zana* matting which was a woven grass. These would be carried on and then taken away to make room for other events.

There would be wrestling displays to entertain us all, and demonstrations by the butchers of how they would bring the huge bulls to the ground in order to control them. The bulls would, I remember, be held at first by two men, one of whom hung on to a rope tied to one of the animal's back legs, while the other grasped a rope tied to the opposite foreleg. The butcher himself would then approach the bull from the front, and holding its horns, would try to turn its head, thus making it lose its balance and fall to the ground. Generally they did this pretty well – except for one occasion when the bull won and gored the butcher. I saw this happen and was able to get him quickly to the hospital where we took him straight into theatre. Luckily the wound, though potentially severe, healed up well and he went home in due course with no lasting harm done.

Another thing shown at this event sometimes was a great lorry piled high with dead quelea birds. This sounds cruel, but these birds, though small and dainty looking, were like feathered locusts in their destructive actions. They would descend in their thousands on crops of grain and within a few hours would eat the whole crop. They were a huge, huge problem. All sorts of methods were devised to try to control them, but the only thing that worked was to destroy them en masse. Lorry loads gave everybody an idea of just how many birds came and ate the grain. Unless you had seen it, you just could not imagine it. One lorry load was only a small part of the season's take.

There was always a huge crowd of spectators at the Agricultural Show – people crammed themselves in to whatever space there was, however small. The neem trees surrounding the arena would be climbed by innumerable small boys and larger youths, as would also be the case at Race Meetings. Every branch would be occupied with at least one lad, sometimes by several, sitting there, legs dangling, enjoying themselves and shouting appropriate comments. Often the trees were actually outside the arena so that no admission fee was paid by their occupants, who of course had very good ringside seats! The Agricultural Show was never without interest.

People often ask me "Did you see many snakes?" I saw very few actually, and would probably have seen more if I'd lived in the river belt. However, I did come across an occasional one, and generally in an odd circumstance. The introductory snake came along when I had only been in Africa for a few weeks. I was lying in my bath one evening, enjoying the chance to relax at the end of a busy day, when suddenly a small green head came through the overflow just under the tap. The head was followed by a long green slender body. Before the whole thing slithered into the water, it stopped and had a good look round. For several seconds the snake and I solemnly regarded one another, each of us, no doubt, wondering what was the best thing to do. The snake blinked first, and as suddenly as it had arrived, it quietly retreated. Hastily I pulled the plug and got out of the bath. It never occurred to me then or later to have a quick look round the house to make sure there were no other thin green snakes anywhere. What could I have done anyway if there were? A month or two later, as I was closing the lounge windows before going to bed, I heard a strange crunching noise. On investigation I found that I had unwittingly killed a snake just as it was coming into the house.

Another time was when I was putting the children's toys away after they had gone to bed. The doors were open on to the verandah where Rex and I would sit for the rest of the evening enjoying the cool air. Just as I had piled the last wooden bricks and soft toys into the basket and was pushing it across the floor to its proper place, out from amongst the contents slid a small black snake which then shot away into the garden. These 'house vipers', as we called them, though their bites would not be fatal in adults, could nevertheless be pretty dangerous for children. That one gave me quite a shock.

The last snake story I will tell happened one morning. While we were having breakfast, we suddenly became aware of a bit of a commotion outside. When I went out to see what was going on, I found our steward and the garden boy dragging a huge spitting cobra into the garden. The garden boy said that he was coming to work when he saw this snake in his path. He managed to find a big stick which he used to kill it. Now they were bringing it to show us. At that time we had a new doctor at the hospital. He was interested in snakes and had asked us all to bring any snakes to him so that he could see what we had in and around Maiduguri.

This will be a good one for him, I thought, and told the boys to put it into the garage saying that when I went back to work after breakfast I would take it to the hospital for the MO to see. Imagine my consternation when I went to the garage to find that the cobra had only, it seemed, been stunned, and was now wriggling round the garage trying to find the way out. It looked enormous, and was, as we discovered after it had been killed again and properly this time, a good six feet long. I was very glad that it had recovered when it did, instead of perhaps waiting until it was in the back of my car and on the way down to the hospital before it regained its senses! I packed it very securely in a big box, just in case, before I drove off.

We thought it had probably come from a group of cobras that lived in a huge tree just outside the compound near the boys' quarters. We had been told about them when we first moved on to the college campus, as they had frequently raided a chicken coop on the next door Craft School compound, so they were already known about. However, they had never bothered any of us – we left them alone, and normally they left us alone. I suppose you could say that my husband and I were no spring chickens, and therefore of no interest to the snakes.

I had been told, when I first arrived in Maiduguri, never to get out of the car, especially at night, without looking at the ground outside the car door, just in case I had stopped next to a snake. I did this religiously to start with, but soon forgot to bother. What I did not forget to do, though, was always to shake my sandals, or any other footwear, in the morning before putting them on, in case a scorpion had decided to take shelter there during the night.

Talking of snakes reminds me quite inconsequentially about bees. African bees were, I am sure, much more fierce than the ones we come across in the

UK. This was brought home to me when one evening I was called to the Nursing Home for an emergency admission and was surprised to be told that three people – father, mother and child – had come along with bee stings. I thought, as I got into the car, that they must be making a bit of a big thing about just a bee sting, but kept an open mind as to what I would find. The Africans never ceased to amaze me with their descriptions of various complaints, and after being told that 'crocodiles in the hair' meant nothing more than head lice, I was prepared for anything at any time. However, when I saw my newly arrived patients, they had indeed been stung by bees – and badly too.

It turned out that this small family, on a long journey, had been well on the road to Maiduguri where they were booked in to the Rest House, when misfortune befell them. They had been driving all morning, and had decided to stop for a rest and to have something to eat and drink en route.

It was the hottest part of the day, and the country through which they were driving was just orchard bush and sandy scrub, with not much in the way of shade. However, they spotted a larger tree a little way from the road, parked the car at the roadside and went to sit down in the shade under the tree while they ate.

In next to no time, however, they found themselves being attacked by hundreds of bees which, unknown to them, must have had a nest in the tree, or been swarming there. The father said that they rolled in the sand to try to rid themselves of the bees, but that all three of them quickly became unconscious. He was the first to recover his senses, to find his wife and child still unconscious near to him – and all three of them were still being stung by angry bees. He started to try to drag his family to the car, but couldn't do much as he was still in a pretty fragile state himself. Luckily just at that moment, some men came by, driving a herd of cattle in front of them. He called to them and several came to help, and they got the mother and child into the car for him, and helped him into it as well. He said that he shut all the car windows and just sat there until he felt a bit better, by which time the other two had recovered consciousness. As soon as he felt able he resumed the journey to Maiduguri, still a hundred or so miles farther on, knowing that at least they had a place booked there where they could sleep overnight, and he hoped that there would be some medical help too, which there was.

I respected African bees after that, and nobody need tell me about 'stirring up hornets' nests' ever again. Hornets must be child's play compared with what happened to these poor souls that day.

Many people would come to the hospital with scorpion stings, of which everyone seemed to be very afraid. I think they expected every scorpion sting to be fatal, but in fact our local variety was not dangerous, luckily, albeit painful at the time. My husband knew about this himself. He had just gone back to the lounge to collect a book to read in bed, and went barefoot. I heard him shout, and ran through to see what was the matter. He was half laughing and half in pain. Apparently while he was walking along, a scorpion had run just in front of him, and had stung him first on one big toe and then on the other as it passed his feet. All he needed was a couple of aspirin tablets and the pain soon subsided. However, all my African patients expected (and I have to say, got) an injection, just one shot, of something we actually used for another specific complaint. It always cured them within minutes and they had great faith in it. Sometimes a little faith healing like that was quicker than trying to explain things – and your explanations wouldn't always be believed anyway.

I have spoken about snakes and insects. You may ask – what about other animals? Well, there must have been some somewhere, but we didn't see very much in station. I have already mentioned baboons and some monkeys that I saw when I was touring. And from time to time one would see small antelopes dart into or from the bush on the roadside.

Generally they simply darted back again if they saw anything moving like a car. But one poor little duiker, an animal like a small deer, was not so lucky. I was driving home one evening up the last stretch of the tree lined road to the GRA when suddenly this small animal bounded out of the shadows of the trees and onto the bonnet of my car where it lay motionless. I stopped the car, but then decided to drive the last hundred yards to my house very slowly with the duiker still on the bonnet, thinking that if it was simply stunned it would have a chance to recover. Sadly it was dead and I asked my house-boys to dispose of it. No doubt they enjoyed bush meat that night. My cook told me afterwards that inside it there had been a baby duiker. One should not mourn over this accident but it did seem sad to think of two little lives lost in such a way.

Once we had a sittatunga in the compound, another deer like animal, with white markings on its sides. Possibly this was a young one because it was quite small. I understood that they liked to live near water but, although normally very shy, this one stayed in our dry compound for several days before disappearing as suddenly as it came.

But generally we saw nothing more. We knew that hyenas lived in the bush, and occasional leopards, but again, one didn't expect to see any of them in station either, well, not as a general rule anyway.

However, shortly after our son was born in 1962, there was a brief period when a leopard did stalk the GRA in Maiduguri. At first there was just a rumour that one had been seen leaping off a roof. Everyone dismissed that as being just a rumour. But then a leopard was indeed seen to be coming in to the station, and in different areas too. One of the expatriate teachers at the Women's Training College, who was by that time sleeping out on her verandah, it being the hot season, found its footprints all over the verandah when she got up in the morning, and from the disturbance of the sandy dust under her bed she realised that it had actually rested there during the night.

At that time we too were sleeping outside. The children's beds were on the verandah while our bed was a few yards away from them out into the compound. Our son was only a few weeks old. I felt rather anxious, thinking that if this animal decided to wander down along the airport road and found all the educational institutions and staff houses there, it could pose problems. What would we do if it came into our compound? How would we get to the children to take them inside? Would they be in danger if we didn't? A small baby would be a tempting morsel for a hungry leopard, I thought. The next day we heard that it had been seen at the Secondary School next door to the college. That decided me, and I had our beds all moved back into the house. Hot or not hot, I thought, we'll just have to endure the heat in order to be safe.

The very next night, I suddenly roused in the small hours, to hear a low grunting sort of a cough somewhere outside. I woke right up. "Leopards cough!" I told myself, and got out of bed and looked out of one of the windows which overlooked the bush at the back of the house. Nothing to be seen there. I went to the glass doors that opened from the bedroom into our compound. Nothing there. But I felt sure that was what I had heard. The next morning when I got up, and when it was still cool before we went to work, I had a look round the compounds. There unmistakeably were great paw tracks in both compounds. The animal must have leapt over a seven foot wall to get in and out, and it must have tracked all round outside the building to reach the walls bounding both our garden areas and explored them both. You could see in the sand where its tail had trailed as it walked across. As the heat increased so the marks on the verandah faded – there must have been some moisture on its paw pads, which had left marks on the paving stones, and which evaporated as the sun got up. But the tracks in the sand remained.

The next night we asked our night watchman if he had seen anything. Yes, he had seen this animal coming towards him, and, as we had suggested he should do if there was any danger, he had quickly climbed into one of our cars and stayed there until the leopard went away. How glad I was that we had moved all our beds back into the house. After that, nobody seemed to see or hear anything of the animal again – perhaps it simply continued up the airport road until it found an area uninhabited by humans where it could live in peace.

And lions? Well, it was said that there had been lions around once, long ago, though not any more. However, an American Aid group came out to build a cattle ranch some little way out of Maiduguri. I think they thought it would provide a more settled life for the wandering Fulani who were the great cattlemen there. But after the ranch had come into being, the odd lion was once more seen in the district, and indeed, some of the cattle were being killed. This was thought, needless to say, to be because the cattle were now static instead of being taken, nomad fashion, to different grazing grounds all the time. We heard that somebody who was interested in hunting was asked to go and help deal with whichever lion had been nicking the cows. He loaded up his vehicle with all the gear, and drove out to the village to do his good deed. Alas, on arrival he was told that they didn't need his help after all because they had hunted the lion themselves and shot and killed it – with their bows and arrows. A disconsolate gentleman returned to station.

Chapter 25

Doctors came and went at all hospitals in Nigeria during the years I was out there. Somebody new was posted in whenever a medical officer went on leave, so the staffing changed every few months or so. Louis had long gone from Maiduguri. He had become very senior and was working in Kaduna. Over the years, as said earlier, I had worked with medical staff of various nationalities: English, German, Czech, Egyptian, Indian, Irish, Malaysian. And shortly before we left Nigeria we had, in Maiduguri, one of the first Nigerian doctors to be trained in his own country as well. I don't know how comprehensive a training he would have had as compared with what I had been given, but he was a hard and willing worker, and a pleasant colleague to have around. In these later years we had a very good Nursing Sister posted to the Nursing Home once we were able to have it open permanently for both inpatients and outpatients. Sister Ibiam, was excellent and I enjoyed working with her.

I often think how interested I would be to see how medical and nursing training have progressed in the North since I left. But the nursing was as yet rather erratic, or could be. The senior staff were pretty good, but the more junior members varied. Partly, I think, this was because the ethos of medical and nursing care was not yet fully understood, but partly, especially with night staff, it was because many would actually be very tired when they came on duty. Most local people did not really cater for people who had to sleep in the day and work at night. There was always a good deal of noise in any household, with people coming and going all the time. The result of this was actually brought home to me at the time of the birth of my second child. I had been settled for the night before the day staff went off duty, and all seemed well. However, during the night I woke and was not as well as I should have been. I rang the bell for the nurse – nobody came. I rang again. Still nobody. I decided that I should get up and try to get down the corridor to see where she was. There was no one about, not in the duty room, not in any of the other cubicles – I was the only patient there. There was nobody in the delivery room, nobody anywhere. I tried to telephone the other MO. No reply from the operator at the exchange either.

I decided that I would just have to cope on my own and returned to my room. Just as I was turning in at the door of my cubicle, I almost tripped over what looked like a bundle of clothes just outside the door. Laundry for tomorrow, I thought, and then suddenly looked again. No, not laundry, but the night nurse, curled up on the floor and fast asleep. At least she had dossed down at my door, imagining no doubt that she would hear me if I called. Well, one of us might as well have a good night, I thought, and I let her sleep on.

The training that many of the nursing staff had, although it was clearly improving all the time, was not as comprehensive as that in the UK. A general idea would catch on, but the reasoning behind the teaching could pass by, so that things were frequently not properly done, though they would be nearly properly done. It would have been counterproductive to carp all the time. For one thing, some staff might be afraid of a telling-off and therefore not be totally upfront about things. It was better to know if things were not perfect, and why, rather than live in an unreal world of thinking that everything was hunky dory. I learnt that if I was prepared within reason to compromise a little, then the people I was working with would find it easier to raise their game and none of us would be upset. That way we achieved a great deal. It was also vital to retain a sense of humour. Without that one might as well pack up and go home. Laughter is a great leveller and a great help – especially being able to laugh at oneself.

At the Provincial Girls' School, the young girl who acted as 'house mother' to them and who helped me in my clinics there, was rather quiet one day and seemed to be a bit down hearted. I asked her if anything was wrong. She told me that she was going to leave her employment there.

"But I thought you were happy here," I said.

"Yes, I am very happy and I don't want to leave. But my family say that I must marry now and not work. I don't want to marry – I want to stay here and work."

"Well, can't you say so to your family?" I asked.

"Dr Abraham, it is different for you," she replied sadly, "In your country women like you who are married can still work, and if you don't want to be married you can stay not married without disgracing your family, and you can still work and it is all right. Already I am old to be marrying, but I have to do it now or disgrace them all."

Meriam (not her real name) was all of about 16 or 17 years old. Poor Meriam. She was such a nice girl and excellent at what she did. The schoolgirls all liked her and she was totally reliable. I never had any anxiety about leaving instructions with her, and if I 'admitted' any of the girls to her sickbay I knew they would be well looked after. I missed her very much when she left, and have often wondered whether, as the years passed, she was able eventually to work again.

The position of women was strange to people like me, in that often they seemed to be very much second class citizens, doing many of the more menial jobs, walking behind their husbands (who often rode horses or donkeys while their wives followed on foot). Particularly in respect of wives from the southern region, some would bring letters with them when they attended the outpatient clinics, written by their husbands or by scribes, setting out their symptoms and complaints. It was as if they would not be capable of speaking for themselves. Other women, both southerners and northerners were well capable of speaking to me directly however, and did so. I think they all appreciated having a woman doctor around the place.

Although women appeared to be subservient, some at least of the Kanuri women had a quite independent attitude. Clearly it helped a lot that I could speak a little Hausa, for this meant that they had no need to go through an interpreter who was often one of our male nurses. But the women who seemed to be far more timid and unable to say anything for themselves were some of the Pakistani and Arab wives. If I was asked to see them, they would more often than not be accompanied by their husbands, who would speak English. I could see the need for this. However, instead of the husband translating my questions so that these women could know what I had asked and could reply themselves, the husbands often simply answered without telling them what I had said. Moreover, if I then wanted to examine any of these women, they were only permitted to reveal about a square inch of body at a time – they could never undress so that I could make a proper examination. It was very awkward at times and one always felt that one might be missing an important clinical finding. But that never changed and I had to do the best I could under those conditions. I supposed it was to do with Islam, but I wished that the husbands had understood how important a proper examination of one's patient could be, and I always worried that I might be missing something. I often wondered too if the women themselves ever wished they could speak directly to me and explain themselves properly.

It often seemed that not only had I to 'make do and mend' in regard to equipment, but also in my dealings with some of these patients. Like I said, you just had to do the best you could, given the circumstances at the time.

There was so much that could have been done in other ways too, given the staff. I felt that if only people understood why we embarked on this or that treatment, and why it was important that they should stick to it properly, and why it was important that they should play their part in regard to life style ... if only, if only. As it was, you barely had time to handle what came your way. You simply could not think of expanding your activities to include teaching sessions. Too many factors worked against what we tried to do in those days.

I have said before, and it should bear repeating, that in station we to had to battle against the fact that people often waited until they were desperately ill before coming to the hospital. This was certainly the case if they lived a long distance away, due to the costs of transport and also seasonal problems with the roads and tracks. And so they would often arrive when little help was possible. In this way they came to associate the hospital with dying. It was hard work persuading people to come early so that there was a better chance of recovery for most patients. The medical officers' bush touring was confined to the dry season and there were not enough of us to get round as often as we would like. Then again, older people in a village, when confronted with new ideas about health, would say firmly, "That is not our custom" and the new ideas would be dismissed.

Our children were growing. They loved having Grace to look after them when I was out, and played happily all day long. They had 'little' friends who came to our house, and were invited back. However, I wondered if we could get some other interest going for them, and when, towards the end of 1963, we were offered the use of an old retired polo pony, it seemed to fill the bill. Dan Tanda (the horse) and Abba (the elderly horse-boy) came up to us two or three times a week, and the little contingent would set off and be out for an hour. Both children would be in the saddle at the same time, and Abba would take the lead. Although Abba often didn't bother to hold the reins when the children were up, Dan Tanda always followed him absolutely. Grace would bring up the rear. In due course they would come back, still going at the same quiet pace. Then (it was always in the afternoon), if I was not busy I would in turn ride out on Dan Tanda for half an hour. He was always very quiet and gentle – until, that is, he saw a games field. As we were in the middle of the Secondary School, the Craft school and the College campuses, we saw a lot of games fields. As soon as he spotted goal posts, Dan Tanda would prick up his ears, gather himself together, and take off. He must have enjoyed polo, for he would gallop like mad right up the field, whether anyone was playing football there or not. At the goalposts, he would stop. He took me by surprise at first, but I learnt to stay away from danger and took him instead out into the bush.

Abba kept the horse beautifully. There was a condition attached to Dan Tanda. He was really quite an elderly animal, and the expatriate who had owned him and who had now retired, had left money for his upkeep and for that of Abba, with the proviso that if he was ridden by anyone but Abba, he must only ever be ridden by a European. He felt that not all Africans would be gentle with a horse (they often were not, and the African bits were not comfortable ones either).

One time when they were out, there was a sudden heavy downpour, it being the rainy season. As the rain didn't stop, I thought I would drive through the Craft School compound to collect Grace and the children and bring them home. I knew that they generally came home that way. I had only got as far as the main entrance to the school when I saw them. It was really one of the funniest sights I'd ever seen. The entrance was a big archway with two wings of the building on either side. The archway was approached by several steps.

The little contingent, horse and all, had climbed the steps, to shelter under the roof of the arch. The children were both up in the saddle, and Grace and Abba stood on either side. While I was there, the rain stopped, and they all descended the stair and proceeded in their usual manner back to our house. I had the crazy feeling that had the headmaster of the Craft School opened his office door and invited them in, they would have walked in there with similar gravity, horse included. Nothing seemed to faze that animal.

During our last few years in Maiduguri, work finally began on the building of the railway between Jos and Maiduguri. This had been planned for a very long time, and indeed, I hadn't long been in Maiduguri on first arrival in 1957 when I attended the ceremony at which the old Shehu had hammered in a stake to show where the railway would end and the station platform would begin. Now, during 1964, I was to see the railway itself being built through virgin bush. It was to pass less than quarter of a mile behind our house, and we were able therefore to see every stage in the process. Years previously I had read and enjoyed a book, in which part of the storyline was the description of the building of a railway. I had found this to be extremely interesting, and as I watched things happening near us, I recognised so much of what I had read in that book. It was actually very helpful, almost as if it had been a textbook!

First of all the trace was built – a high ridge with a flat top on which the actual lines would be laid. Later we saw the lines and wooden sleepers being put down. The walk to the railway became a regular short trip after siesta for us all. It wasn't too far for the children, and Rex and I were both keen to see how it was getting on, so we would all four amble across the bush once or twice a week to have a look. Gradually it all took shape, though I wondered often how stable those lines would be when heavy trains ran over them – they had seemed more like toys when they were being put down – a sort of grown-up Meccano.

But at last, after many months, the first engine was to be sent up the line. This would be a great day, we thought, and the four of us went along to see it. For several minutes nothing happened – then, in the far distance we saw a faint plume of smoke. It got bigger and blacker, and finally we saw the engine, still far away, looking like a little toy Hornby engine coming along. It travelled very slowly, and then, rather disappointingly, stopped about a hundred yards short of where we stood. I had just time to take a photograph of it, before it reversed and went back, disappearing into the distance once more. Still, so far, so good. At least the line was OK up to where the engine stopped, and we felt that we had seen a bit of history in the making.

We ourselves were never to see the first train into Maiduguri however, but we were told by friends that, when it did come, the local people were so excited to see a train – something that most were looking at for the first time ever – that many had rushed on to the line, trying to touch the engine to see what it felt like. Some were injured, needless to say. My husband had once been posted to Gombe where a railway had also been built. He often said to me that where a railway went, so too would go more thieves, as everyone had discovered. He predicted that this could happen in Maiduguri as well.

And so the days and months passed. Rex and I would sit on the verandah before going to work early in the morning, drinking tea, and listening to a hornbill's strange call as it sat every day at the same time in a nearby tree, stretching its neck and flapping its wings as it squawked. I would try to dash home mid morning to make sure everything was all right with the children before I went to the Nursing Home to do a Senior Service surgery there, after which I would continue with the school work until lunch time.

Once a week, just before lunch, I would do my big weekly shopping at one of the canteens. Usually I went to Chellaram's, an Indian canteen along the Avenue of the Sudan, rather separated from the others on the Maiduguri 'beach'. It was a very good canteen and, being forward looking, was run on the lines of our present day supermarkets – we went round, loading our containers with goods which we then paid for at a cash desk – the first time I had ever seen this system.

Nobody knew the full name of one of the two Indian managers there – we only ever knew his first name which was Rai, so we all called him 'Rai Chellaram'. He was a very matter of fact individual, also very kind and hospitable, having many of us for dinner at his house from time to time. I remember how once when several of us were at his house, the conversation turned to game reserves. There was a reserve a hundred miles or so from Maiduguri to which quite a number of people from the station would go for a spot of local leave. "Have you ever been, Rai?" somebody asked him, "There are all sorts of animals there, lions, giraffe, elephants." Rai chuckled. "Why would I want to go all that way to see elephants?" he asked, "I had a whole line of elephants at my wedding!"

Things in Maiduguri were changing following Independence. The last British Resident, Nicky McClintock, had gone and had been replaced by a Nigerian Provincial Commissioner who lived in the Residency where I had stayed just before my wedding. That too had now changed, and the original

232

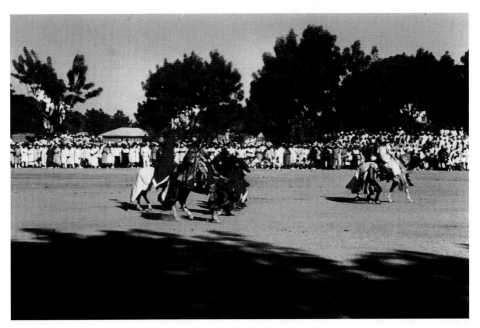

Caparisoned horses at a durbar in Maiduguri, c. 1960. See the spectators in the trees.

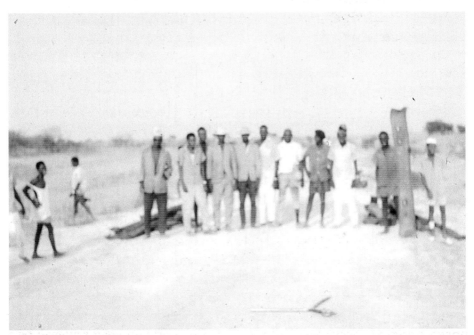

Workers prepare to lay the first sleepers on the newly built railway trace near Maiduguri, 1963-4.

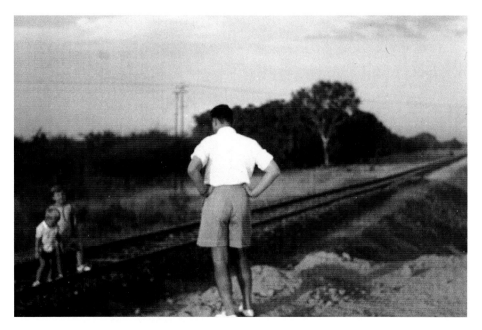

Rex and the children looking at the newly completed railway line, 1964. As yet it was not in use and no train had been on it.

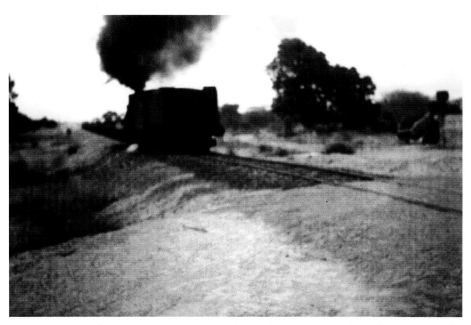

Later in 1964 the first engine to travel on the Bornu railway line chugged slowly to a point near the Bornu Training College, stopped for a few moments, and then, as shown here, chugged just as slowly all the way back again.

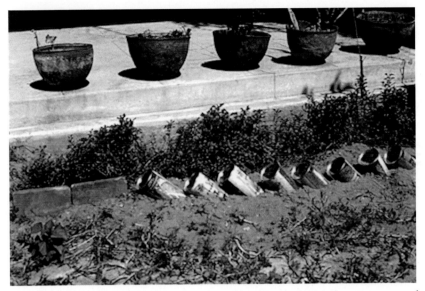

The garden boy had his own ideas about beautifying the compound round our house.

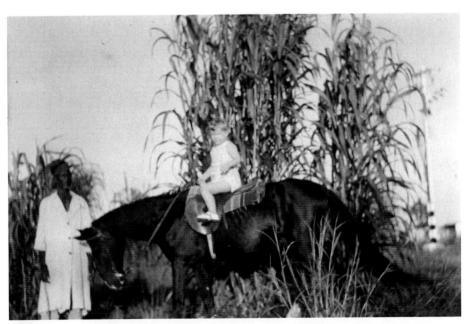

Abba the horse boy, Dan Tanda the horse, and Rosemary our daughter, 1964.

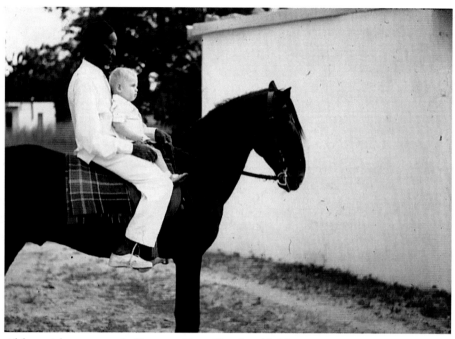

Abba with our son Julian on Dan Tanda, 1964.

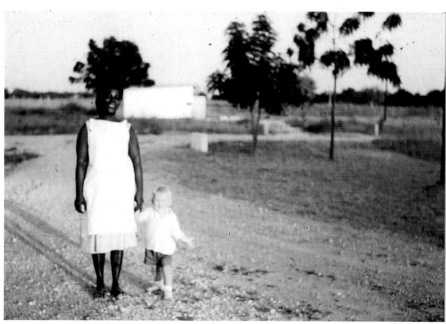

Grace with Julian, 1964.

servants' quarters now seemed to be the living accommodation for his wives, while only the Commissioner lived in the house as far as I could make out. It had been a surprise to me when I was asked to visit one of the wives because she was not well, to be redirected from the house to what I had known as the boys' quarters. I suppose that the wives would not be expected to appear in public, or at least would not be expected to take any prominent part in official functions, though they would be allowed to sit in the background at events like durbars. I never formally met any of the Emir of Katsina's wives on official occasions even though they might be there in the background, although as I have said, I went often to their compound and sat amongst them and their children, and found them to be a jolly lot. The Provincial Commissioner himself would have many duties, and would often have to provide hospitality for important visitors, which would mean using all the rooms in the Residency.

The Southern Nigerians were different, and my impression was that Southern wives took a much bigger part in family affairs and had more independence. Well, many of them did. When word got round that we were leaving Nigeria on final retirement, I was invited (on my own and at different times) by several Southern wives in the town to visit and enjoy a cup of tea with them as a sort of farewell. I didn't know most of them, but it seemed that I had seen them as patients, and I found it interesting to visit the different African households. Our children had been invited to the odd birthday party organised by Southern families too.

At our wedding reception, we had been taken a little by surprise when two unexpected guests had appeared in the line to shake hands with us. They were also Southerners, a husband and wife who ran a little shop just near the hospital. Their shop was where Rex and I had often popped in to buy cans of cold Fanta Orange, which they had started to stock and which we had not seen anywhere else. Because they didn't have ice or a refrigerator in the shop, the cans were kept in a tank of water so that evaporation would cool them. The news of our engagement and marriage must have got round to them, so they came to the wedding and the reception. Perhaps they were members of the church. We didn't know, but we were pleased that they had come along. Although we had several other Africans on that occasion, people who we had invited, they were all northerners and not one brought his wife with him. A complete difference.

Another change that came about was the tarring of the road from Bauchi to Maiduguri. When I had first arrived, only the road from Jos to Bauchi was tarred. Now the whole lot was dealt with. It took several months, but gradually the work was done. Workers of all nationalities were drafted in. One of our friends on the station was an Indian civil engineer, who, after long hours of surveying in the heat, would come round in the evenings sometimes for a chat and a long cool drink, and would say wearily, "I have been chaining the road all day." It would have been hot work for all the people on that project. Quite a number of Italians were engaged on the road building too. I always thought of the tremendous road making achievements of the Ancient Romans and thought what I was seeing in Nigeria was history repeating itself.

The college grew so much that we no longer knew each student like we had known the first class or even the second and third year's intake. There were now so many students that increasing numbers had to live in the town. The existing dormitories were full, and conversations were being held with the Maiduguri Native Authority to see whether designated student accommodation could be made available in the town. There was no way in which we could invite a group to our house for tea occasionally as we had once done. A flourishing establishment can sometimes be so big, I suppose, that although it gains by its success, its very size means that something is also lost.

The expatriate medical and nursing staff at the Maiduguri General Hospital had changed many times since I first went there. Louis had been promoted a year or two before, and was now very senior and working on the admin side at the Ministry of Health in Kaduna.

The Waziri of Bornu, Shettima Kashim Ibrahim, was no longer based in Maiduguri, having been made the first Nigerian Governor of the Northern Region. He had also been knighted and was now Sir Kashim Ibrahim. He was well liked by the expatriate community. He had a dry sense of humour which I always enjoyed. I still have the gift he sent to us for our marriage. Happily he kept on his house in Maiduguri (now referred to as his 'Maiduguri Lodge') and when in town he hosted lunch parties to which several of us would be invited.

With the coming of Independence the permanent service officers (expatriates) realised that their futures had to be carefully considered. Those of us who had heard the Sardauna of Sokoto speaking in 1957 to expatriate heads of department remembered how he had said, "After Independence we will continue to employ you for as long as we want you, but when the time comes for you to go, you will go."

We all knew that the older one was, the harder it would be to get decent employment on return to our own countries. No more permanent expatriate officers were being taken on in Northern Nigeria – new people coming were all on contract now. Some of the permanent people were starting to think of retiring from the service while they were still young enough to find work back home. Others decided to stay on no matter what.

British expatriate officers in permanent service posts who decided to leave the service while still under retirement age were offered various options to compensate for loss of career. These options included either pension arrangements or offers of equivalent posts in other colonies.

For instance, at that time, among the list of possible appointments that we saw, there was mention of two jobs going in, I think, Fiji, where they wanted both an education officer and a medical officer. Had we wanted to work overseas again, that combination would have suited us very well.

Back in early 1962 my husband and I had already been thinking about all this. As a permanent service officer, Rex had by then given ten years of his working life to service in Nigeria. He had worked his way up from Education Officer through the ranks of seniority and different education disciplines (and would, in fact, be promoted in 1963 to Principal Education Officer, though he didn't yet know about that). Finally he had been given his own college to run, building it up from its first class in poor accommodation to its present size and on its own extensive campus. It had become a flourishing establishment. Everything about it – its ethos, the uniforms, the college crest, the format of each day, the harmony between the various religions of the students, staff relationships – all these things had been worked out by him from the start, and he was now seeing the results of his efforts. He loved the work and had put his heart and soul into it. It was heartbreaking to think of perhaps leaving everything he had done now.

I too, realised what a wrench it would be for me to leave Nigeria. Having 'done time' as a general medical officer with hospital and touring work, I was now still building up my school medical service and had ideas about how it could be extended if I could get more help. As yet this service had really only just been born and there was a lot that could be done given the facilities. And I was still managing to do bits of hospital and Nursing Home duties as well. I enjoyed every minute of it all, demanding though it was.

In the end however, fate, as so often happens, stepped in. It transpired that the Ford Foundation of America and American Aid were to finance a scheme to assist selected training colleges in Northern Nigeria. They intended sending a team of tutors from Wisconsin University to Nigeria, as well as providing funds for classrooms and other facilities in the college or colleges selected. The scheme was to start in January 1965. With this in mind, in January 1964 somebody from the Ford Foundation together with a professor from Wisconsin University came to Nigeria to look at the colleges there in order to make a decision. In due course they came to Maiduguri and looked at the Bornu Training College. They talked at length to Rex about their plans and ideas. And they selected Bornu Training College for their scheme. This was a feather in Rex's cap, for his was not the only men's teacher training college in the North by any means. He was pressed to stay on to work with the Wisconsin team, although he was told, "We are aware of the decisions you are having to make about your career now that Nigeria is fully independent, and we can't offer you anything with us after we leave here."

In the end, Rex felt that he didn't want to stay on and see his college perhaps being – in the nicest possible way – 'over run' by a large group of people all at once, none of whom knew anything about Nigeria and Nigerians. New members of expatriate staff could, and did, come to the college quite often. But they came in small enough numbers, only one or two at a time, to be gradually integrated as they learnt to understand the country and the students. A large group of people, coming all at one time, probably with their own ideas and fact-finding zeal could, he felt, have the potential to upset other staff members, though he hoped it wouldn't be like that. But he felt more and more, and with great sadness, that he did not want to stay and see his college, his 'baby', perhaps change in ways that he was not happy about. Moreover, our first child was just coming up to school age. There was no school for her in Maiduguri, and if Rex stayed on we would inevitably have had to separate for many months at a time to fit in with school terms in the UK. Neither of us wanted that, so we finally accepted that the time had come to leave Nigeria. We gave notice that we would proceed on retirement from the Service at the end of 1964. And so the die was cast.

For my part, there were still things – not all of them connected with my work, that I had not been able to do during my years overseas. I had not, for instance, ever managed to get to Lake Chad. Even at the very last minute, when we were in the throes of organising our departure, an invitation had been extended to me: transport, accommodation and two or three days at the Lake with the chance to go out on one of the reed boats which were made and used by the local fishermen there, a trip that Rex had made when on tour as PEO some years earlier. However, I could not have left the children, and in any case by that time I was well occupied with packing, finishing off my professional tasks and so on. I had to refuse that last chance.

We had never managed to visit the game reserve, which we had all wanted so much to see. I had not seen Fort Lamy – the capital of Chad, where most people tried to get to for a few days' local leave, and where there were good shops, and where the stewards at the hotel were flamboyant in wide Zouave trousers.

I had had to pass up on a chance to go to Timbuktu as well, when we were in Katsina. One of the nursing sisters had worked out that it would be possible from Katsina to get to Timbuktu quite easily – it would have meant a longish drive to the Niger, a river trip, and a final drive from there, but it could be done. She wanted to have a go. Would I be interested? Well, of

236

course I would – but by that time I had a baby of only one or two months old. It was just not possible for me either to take an infant on such a trip, or to leave her at home if I went. So no Timbuktu for me either. Well, those were all places I must continue to dream about. I had, after all, enjoyed a life of immense interest as it was, and would have much to remember in later years.

Chapter 26

There was still much to do before we left – in any case there was a long period of notice to serve before we would go, together with all sorts of prior administrative processes to be gone through as well. Rex wanted to make sure that every 't' was crossed and every 'i' dotted in regard to the college before he left it, so that he could hand over as perfect an institution as possible to the incoming Principal. Mr Ita, the chief clerk, was the ideal man to have in that position, and assisted my husband wonderfully well.

Every last detail was checked, and in the last weeks, very comprehensive handing-over notes were compiled and typed out. The last annual speech of the current Principal, including the report on the previous year in the college's life, was put together. Timetables were doubly checked, as were all equipment and stores. The games fields were given a good going-over so that they would be in tip-top condition. Everything was to be left point-device.

But nothing ever goes quite to plan. One morning, just when everything was thought to be as good as you can get, there was a fire in one of the dormitories. The tutor responsible for fire drills went into action, sounding the alarm (a loud whistle), and the students were evacuated from the buildings. The next bit is typical Africa, I think – certainly typical Maiduguri. A phone call was made to call the local Fire Service (one small appliance and a few men). However, the Telephone Exchange operator, through whom all calls had to be made, did not answer the phone for some considerable time, during which the students did what they could with buckets of water. Eventually, with the fire by now burning away merrily, the Fire Service appliance arrived, only to find that just as it arrived, all the water supplies had been turned off, as was normal for that time of day in Maiduguri.

Somehow or other, the fire was extinguished, but a fair amount of damage was done to the dormitory in the meantime. It was thought, after investigation, that an electrical fault had been the cause, so at least it hadn't been student pranks or carelessness.

Nevertheless the procedure after an event like this was that an official Board of Enquiry had to be convened. This meant that somebody from the Ministry of Education in Kaduna had to travel to the college, and the Provincial Commissioner had to attend, as had some of the Native Authority Education officers. It was all such a pity, right at the end of the Rex's time at the college, and especially after all he had done to leave everything in a good state. And it was just one extra time consuming task to take on board when by now we had our sailing date and therefore a deadline for getting everything finished.

During that last year, the college had hosted the Shillingford Sports - these were intercollegiate competitions, when students from all over the North were brought together to take part in athletics, football and other similar activities. A different college was host each time, once it was considered worthy of the task. It was a matter of pride to us in Bornu that the college had achieved that sort of status. Many of the visiting students were from different tribes, and on the whole they were stockier of build and heavier than our young men, who tended to be rather more slender. We thought that at first the outsiders looked with slight contempt at our chaps - until, that is, one was heard to say, after his team lost several running races, "*Kai!* These skinny Bornu boys can run!" Ours were regarded with a lot more respect after that.

Rex had achieved a great deal since he arrived back in Maiduguri to take on the first class of the college. The original thirty students, who squashed themselves, their beds and lockers and all their possessions into one small classroom of a tiny primary school, had long qualified and gone to teach in other junior primary schools all over the province. They had been a nice lot of lads, and had pulled together, I am sure, with much pride, as they saw their college develop into a successful outfit in its large campus. Now we had about three hundred aspiring teachers on the register, smartly turned out at all times and with a sense of belonging to a college which had become both well known and well thought of.

Instead of just one tutor who was also the Principal, there were now thirteen, including American Peace Corps and English Voluntary Service Overseas volunteers. Between them the staff hailed from several countries - England, Nigeria, New Zealand, America, India and Pakistan, and all got on well together. Yes, the first Principal of the Bornu Training College certainly had something to look back on with feelings of great satisfaction.

I too wanted to leave my 'department' in good nick, so that if anyone ever took over an up and running school medical service (unlikely, I knew), there would be something on paper to show what had been done during the last few years. I started to write up my last reports and sent them off to Kaduna, wondering idly if anyone ever read them. I tried to guide the people who had helped in the school clinics so that they would have some sort of structure to work on, though I knew that within hours of my last clinic, the students and school children would once again be trailing down to the hospital, thereby losing hours of classroom time again.

And I began on the all too familiar task of packing up our possessions, this

239

time not just for storage during our leave, but for shipping back to England. I had always done this gradually, so that our house looked much as usual for as long as possible before we vacated it. We also managed to find a good home for Fauna, the little grey cat which, alone of all our pets, had survived the years with us, and had been part of the household. We thought it would be cruel to take him from the tropics straight into a harsh English winter.

I sent away for knitting needles, patterns and wool and began to make sweaters for the children and for us as well. How hot that wool felt to work with in the tropical climate, but I knew that I had to persist, for we would arrive in England in early January when it would be cold. We would be glad of warm wool sweaters then. The only people I had ever seen knitting in Nigeria were the men, funnily enough – I never saw a woman knit, but the men did quite often.

Our cook, Ali, a deeply thinking man, was very anxious about the future. It had not been so very long since the blood bath in the Congo following its independence, and Ali feared that the same thing might happen in Nigeria. "When all the Europeans have gone from Nigeria," he told us rather sadly, "There will be blood here too." He said that many other people in Maiduguri thought the same.

We looked for other employment for our boys so that they would not be without jobs after we had gone. Ali, in fact, got himself a post at the Catering Rest House, so we knew he would be all right, and we managed to find a berth as junior steward for Alamdu, who had been well trained by Ali. The garden boy and our old night watchman as well as Grace, also had new jobs waiting for them when we went.

In order to save a lot of fuss in the Customs Shed in Lagos, I asked the Customs Officer in Maiduguri (for we had a Customs Post, being one of the ports of exit for pilgrims for Mecca) – if he could check and seal all our heavy crates and boxes once they were packed, so that they could go straight through to the ship. Yes, he could and did, coming a day or so before we closed the house, taking a few things out of each box so that he could see what was there before letting me re-pack them tidily. Then he put steel bands round each one and sealed everything with the Customs special seal. This left us with only suitcases and (inevitably) many odd bundles and packages that would travel with us. We were being given many leaving gifts by now, and one never knew what would turn up each day to be packed somehow and taken with us. Farewell parties were being held for us too, and we seemed to be involved with something nearly all the time.

The college staff gave a dinner party, which was held in the college library. It was a lovely occasion, and we enjoyed it enormously, sharing this event with one of the American Peace Corps staff who was also leaving the college.

The hospital staff gave a 'Send-off' party for me, to which Rex was also invited. This was a more formal occasion, with speeches first, followed by dancing, which 'the guest of honour must lead', so I led off, dancing with one of the senior nurses who had acted as chairman for the speeches part of the event. The Medical Social Club, to which all hospital staff belonged, arranged for a big group photograph that included me. It is fun looking at it so many years afterwards, and remembering this or that nurse, the hospital driver, the messenger, and other staff.

The college students and the hospital staff also organised a football match in our honour – which I was asked to start by taking the kick-off (much to my husband's amusement!). At this event too, we were each presented with an outfit of native dress. Rex had a *riga* – the voluminous gown worn by the men, much bigger than a caftan – which he put on over his suit (they excused him from stripping off in order to wear the wide Muslim trousers), and an embroidered cap, the *hula*. Meanwhile, I was taken aside by the women who first pulled a small bodice on to me (again over my dress, so it was all very hot and tight), then for the skirt, wrapped two lengths of cloth round me to cover me from the waist down to my ankles. They finished up by putting a head scarf on me like those that they all wore. These gifts of clothes were very special to us, Rex's outfit being presented to him by his students, and mine by the hospital staff.

We were given bundles of feather fans of all sizes, coloured leather bags and other leather goods, brass ornaments, dishes made of woven grasses, all sorts, and it was quite a problem packing them so that they could be carried. But we felt very touched to be given so much, and from so many different people. It was hard to have to say goodbye.

The day came at last when we handed over the keys of our house and moved into the Rest House for our last two nights. Both Rex and I still had one or two small tasks to finalise the next day, then after a final night, we would be off. The next morning, to our surprise, Grace arrived as usual, saying that she would look after "her *piccins*" (children) for one last day. It was nice of her and a great help to me in fact. I was also by that time being pursued by various people who wanted me to see them professionally before I went, but regretfully I had to say that they must go to the hospital or nursing home as I simply had not got the time to do anything more.

To our surprise too, shortly after Grace had arrived, Abba also appeared, riding Dan Tanda into the Rest House compound. The horse shone like satin, and his hooves positively sparkled – he had been groomed within an inch of his life, while Abba was dressed in his best – a spotlessly white caftan. He too had come to say his goodbyes to us. He chatted to us for a few moments, and then shook hands with us both. He said goodbye – "*Sannu, sai an jima*" – and then suddenly put his head down against the horse's flank. "The English all done go," he said sadly, "What go happen for Nigeria after?" He too was worried about the future now that the expatriates were beginning to leave. Then he remounted and rode away. I don't think our children realised they had seen him for the last time.

At the end of the day Grace, too, left us. I took her down to the town in the car, with the children in the back. When we stopped to let her get out, she turned to my small daughter and spoke to her very seriously, telling her that she must always be a good girl and help her mother, and that when she grew up she must 'find herself a good man' to marry, and that she should be a faithful wife to him. Then she turned to my little son, who was not yet three years old, and she told him that he was to try to grow into a big man and look after his family well. Then, in tears she hugged and kissed them both before getting out of the car.

"Mummy, what was Grace talking about?" asked my daughter wonderingly. Both children were of course far too young to understand what Grace was trying to tell them.

We had planned our journey to Lagos in stages, the first stop being in Kano, where we booked in at the Central Hotel. While we were there, our daughter suddenly said to me, "Will you take me to see that hospital where I was born? I won't ever see it again." I was surprised to hear her ask this – she was only just coming up to five years old. But I took her, as she wished, to Nassarawa Hospital, where she stood for a time in the compound looking very solemnly at the building before she turned to get back into the car.

We drove on the next day to Kaduna, and from there to Ilorin and finally to Lagos. And en route, at last I saw the Jebba Bridge, an impressive structure that spanned the great Niger River. I had missed any sighting of the bridge on my original journey up country by train some seven years previously, because we had crossed it during the night when I was asleep. Having heard about it then, I had been disappointed not to have seen it. This time, as well as slowing down to admire the bridge, we were stopped by soldiers with guns who searched the car before we were allowed to drive on. We couldn't think what the problem was, but perhaps even then there was something in the air akin to unrest, for it was not so very long after we left that we heard of the first uprising before the civil war started.

As we drove on, the landscape altered from orchard bush to great forest trees, where it was quite dark and often felt a bit spooky, I thought.

And at the end of the last long day's drive, we came to Lagos, where we were to stay with a friend overnight before embarking on Elder Dempster's 'Accra' the next morning.

It was very near to Christmas, and our friend had invited one or two other people in for dinner that night and had organised a Christmas meal for us. We all sat round the table and the food was brought in. There was a huge roast turkey, which the steward set down in front of our friend. With a mock shudder, he said, "I can't carve! Put it in front of the lady," and to me he said, "You're the surgeon – get on with it!" So the last bit of knife work I ever did in Nigeria was to carve a Christmas turkey.

The next morning we loaded up the car yet again, packed the children in to what space was left (not very much), and set off for Apapa Wharf. It was my turn to drive, but as neither Rex nor I knew Lagos and its roads it made no difference which of us was at the wheel. We got over the Carter Bridge easily enough, but then were plunged into the horrendous Lagos traffic – cars and vehicles of all sorts everywhere, going in every direction possible. I was disconcerted to say the least when at one moment a double-decker bus mounted the pavement on my near side in order to pass me, and then bounced back down onto the road in front, almost catching my bumper. I was soon completely lost. Somehow I managed to pull in to the side of the busy road, and tried to think what would be the best thing to do. Time was getting on and we had to get to the ship.

Two men walked by just at that moment, and my husband called over to them to ask for directions. "We will do better than tell you," they said, "If you can get us into your car we will go with you and make sure you get there because the way is complicated."

Get them into the car? There wasn't a smidgeon of space left what with luggage and children and us. But "Oh yes, we can both get in here," they said – and one climbed into the back seat amongst all the paraphernalia there, putting our son onto his knee, while the other got into the front (we had a car with a long bench seat at the front), while Rex squashed up nearer to me and took our daughter onto his knee, and somehow we were four adults and two children, all packed into our Citroen Confort amongst the baggage. We were very grateful for their help, for they had us by the ship's side in no time. Wishing us a safe journey and with much shaking of hands (and I think a small financial recompense from my husband), they departed and we embarked, first seeing the car swung up and into the hold. It was December 22nd 1964, just three days before Christmas. We would spend Christmas and New Year on board during the fortnight's voyage to England.

We settled into our family cabin and unpacked what we needed to make it our home for the next two weeks, and then took the children up on deck to explore. They – and we – were delighted to find that there was a supervised nursery where they could play safely. While they were thus occupied, Rex and I stood looking over the side as the ship, already prepared for sailing, cast off and we began to move.

Slowly the West African coast receded as we put out to sea, and I felt an overwhelming sadness for what we were leaving behind.

Nigeria had been a place where a great deal of importance had happened in my life. I'd had a wonderful job, full and satisfying, albeit often frustrating. My whole professional life has been a totally happy one, but I think the years spent in Nigeria were the happiest of all.

In addition to my work in Nigeria, I had met and married Rex and our two children had been born there. Neither Rex nor I had really wanted to leave – we were both committed to our jobs, we both loved the life there and the people amongst whom we worked, but circumstances had made our decision to go inevitable.

I thought back to my first arrival, when I was professionally already pretty experienced but with as yet no knowledge of this new country, its people and culture, or of the system and milieu in which I was to work. My learning curve had been steep as I gradually adjusted in the early months to the many different customs, attitudes and behaviours, as well as to the lack of technical know-how. What a lot I had learnt in the years between, not only about those aspects, but also about myself. And what a lot there was still to be learnt, which I would now never have a chance of doing.

I had never been aware in Nigeria of what people in the UK at that time called 'the colour bar' but which people now call 'racism', and I had never felt any antagonism towards me. I had related to those with whom I worked in the same way as I had done with colleagues in Britain. I had been welcomed into African households and into households of other nationalities as well. The fact that some hospital staff would – and did – pull my leg made me feel that I was accepted for myself and not just because I was 'the doctor'. And indeed, after we were back in England, I sometimes had to think before I remembered if a particular colleague was African or from any other country – we were all just people who worked together. Now we were leaving. I knew that we would never go back.

As we drew farther and farther away and the coastline became fainter, my sadness became unbearable and I went down to the cabin, where Rex, when he came to look for me, found me in tears.

And afterwards?

Still only in our early forties, we had to continue to earn a living. There were many years to go before final pension time.

Rex went into Teacher Training, and I, once the children were both at school, also returned to work, first part time and later, full time. However, instead of going back into hospital work, I went into Community Health because the hours fitted in with our family life. We both managed to climb up the ladder into reasonably senior posts over the next few years. And there we both stayed until our final retirement.

From time to time we had snippets of news of people we had known and worked with. At first we had letters, often written by scribes, from ex employees – Grace, for instance, and our *mai gardi* (night watchman), asking for money or clothing to be sent to them, as well as giving us news about themselves. We had several long and informative letters from Mr Ita, the college clerk, asking after us all and describing the progress of the college through the months after we left. Mr Ita was posted elsewhere himself eventually. I am sure he would give, as always, excellent service wherever he was. Sadly we heard some years later that he had died.

Grace, he told us, eventually moved back to 'her own country', which I think was Calabar, though he didn't have an address for her. We heard no more of her after that.

Ali, our trusted and respected cook-steward, wrote to us a few times, telling us of his family. He and Asumi his wife had one more child, a little girl, who, Ali said, died when only two days old. A friend of ours who had stayed on, told us that Ali was employed at the Maiduguri Catering Rest House, so we knew that he had a regular job after we left Nigeria. Some twenty or so years later, our friend wrote to tell us that Ali too had died. He must have been in his fifties by then.

One or two members of the college staff wrote to my husband at first, the Arabist, for instance, telling of his success in passing some more exams so that he hoped to be able to go on to take a degree. Several of his past students also wrote for a time, telling us the latest college news. Somebody sent us a copy of the student magazine. An interesting development was the setting up of a student court, with the head student acting as 'judge' in the event of misdemeanours. Another new thing was the granting of 'licences' to students who wished to smoke. If any student was caught smoking without a licence, he was fined, quite heavily.

But in the end, the letters stopped as almost always happens. Perhaps it was as well. As I had feared, my school medical service died, I was told, the day after I left, and things reverted to the old pattern of pupils and students missing hours of teaching time because of trailing down to the hospital. I wonder if it ever started up again.

Not long after our return to England, the first uprisings happened in the Northern Region. The Sardauna of Sokoto, who had performed the official opening of the college, was assassinated, as were a number of other people of importance. Northerners and Southerners were pitted against one another and feelings and actions ran high.

We were told later that St John's Anglican Church, where we had been married, had been badly damaged during that time.

Mr Ita, that 'very decent somebody' and his family, he told us afterwards, were taken into the Maiduguri Prison for their own safety. Mr Ita said what a dreadful thing it was to have to be in a prison – I think he didn't like saying where he had been, while at the same time being very grateful to come out of it all alive.

Many houseboys and their families were from the south. A lot of them fled in terror, hoping to be able to get safely to their own regions. Others tried to hide. One of our English friends told us how he hid his steward together with the steward's wife and children, up in the roof space of his bungalow, thus leaving the boys' quarters empty. Our friend told us how unbelievably quiet that little family had managed to be "even the tiny children", during daylight hours, and how they had emerged only once darkness fell, to eat, drink and wash before returning to the roof space before dawn broke. It must have been a truly horrendous time.

Later still, when the subsequent civil war was over and things settled down again in Maiduguri, we heard that permission to hold Sunday services in the little courthouse on the GRA had been withdrawn, so that it could no longer be used as a church.

We also heard that roads which had been named for some of the early explorers, Barth Avenue, Oudney Road, Clapperton Way, Hewby Road and so on, had been given new names. That saddened me, because some of those people had done a lot of good for the Nigerians – without Hewby for instance, who had been the first Resident for Bornu, there might have been no good road down to Biu until long after his time. We were told that The Avenue of the Sudan, that tree lined and sandy road along which I had driven so often to Chellaram's canteen, and along which both Rex and I had driven to the small primary school which originally housed the first class of the college, was also re-named.

Our greatly loved friend and one time colleague, Louis Gonzalez, stayed on in Nigeria for a little longer than we did before retiring to live in Newmarket, where he, like me, went into Community Health. We all kept in touch regularly and he came to stay with us from time to time, before his letters suddenly stopped and somebody we did not know wrote to tell us of his death.

Those of us who remain of the circle of friends from our Nigeria days continue to keep in touch and exchange memories. But the circle grows smaller now. We who worked in pre-Independence Nigeria, and during the early post-Independence years, have, I think, been very privileged to have done so. We all worked hard and most grew to love the country and its people despite the many difficulties and frustrations and the ever-present corruption that permeated all walks of life. I like to think that we all considered ourselves to be 'ambassadors' for our own country and tried to be seen to be 'decent somebodies'.

Although corruption was a way of life among many – not all by any means – of the indigenous people, I think the expatriates were respected and trusted because we were not part of it. Relations between us and those amongst whom we worked were, so far as I am concerned, of the best. We did not interfere with each other's private lives, yet we could and did, socialise in many ways and found plenty of common ground without upsetting each others' culture.

From time to time I look through the things we brought home with us when we retired from overseas service. There are letters, copies of reports in respect of the Bornu Training College and the School Medical Service. There are personal records, bills, receipts, even some of my old Barclays Bank DCO statements. There are photographs and other mementoes – trinkets, fans, leatherwork, brass ornaments, small ivory items and so on.

There are memories too, that take me back to Nigeria. I remember the high pitched whine of the mosquitoes that came as soon as darkness fell. I remember the crowds waiting for me to arrive at the outpatient clinics in the hospitals, and the equally crowded wards with beds and mattresses and sleeping mats all cheek by jowl inside, and out on the verandahs. I remember my limited attempts at Hausa – attempts that nevertheless enabled me to communicate directly with patients, even though they might chuckle at what I was saying. There are memories of Club nights, of music from of the town coming across the warm night air. I hear again the sounds of the market places. I see myself once more at the local race meetings, or the Agricultural Shows. I conjure up the mesmerising sights and sounds of the durbars, with their colours and the jingling of the horses' trappings as they gallop at full speed, kicking up clouds of dust as they go. I call to mind the strains of 'Lilliburlero' that we heard when we turned on our little radio to the BBC Overseas Service to catch a bit of news, or, importantly for Rex, the football commentary from the UK on Saturday afternoons. There are the letters that some of us exchange at Christmas each year with their reminders of our overseas life. And there is always that never-to-be-forgotten memory of the smell of a myriad things – of heat, sand, animals, earth, vegetation, wet dust after rain, people, the smoke of a thousand cooking fires – the smell of Africa as it came over the sea to me when I travelled out there for the first time in 1957.

At such times, it seems important to write down everything I can remember of my years in Northern Nigeria.

However, I am always conscious of the fact that, compared with what countless others had done overseas, my work was really only a very small part. I had spent nothing like the number of years there that many others had done, and I still had much to learn about Nigeria when I finally came back to the UK. It seems presumptuous to be writing this book when I know that many could write far more. It seems sheer cheek to be describing some of the medical tasks that I coped with when I know that other doctors out there tackled far more complex situations. And it is therefore with humility that I have written this at all.

My husband died in 1994.

We never went back.

Greetings, Northern Nigeria, and goodbye.
Sannu – Sai an jima.